Vessel Sanitation Program
2011 Construction Guidelines

I0482665

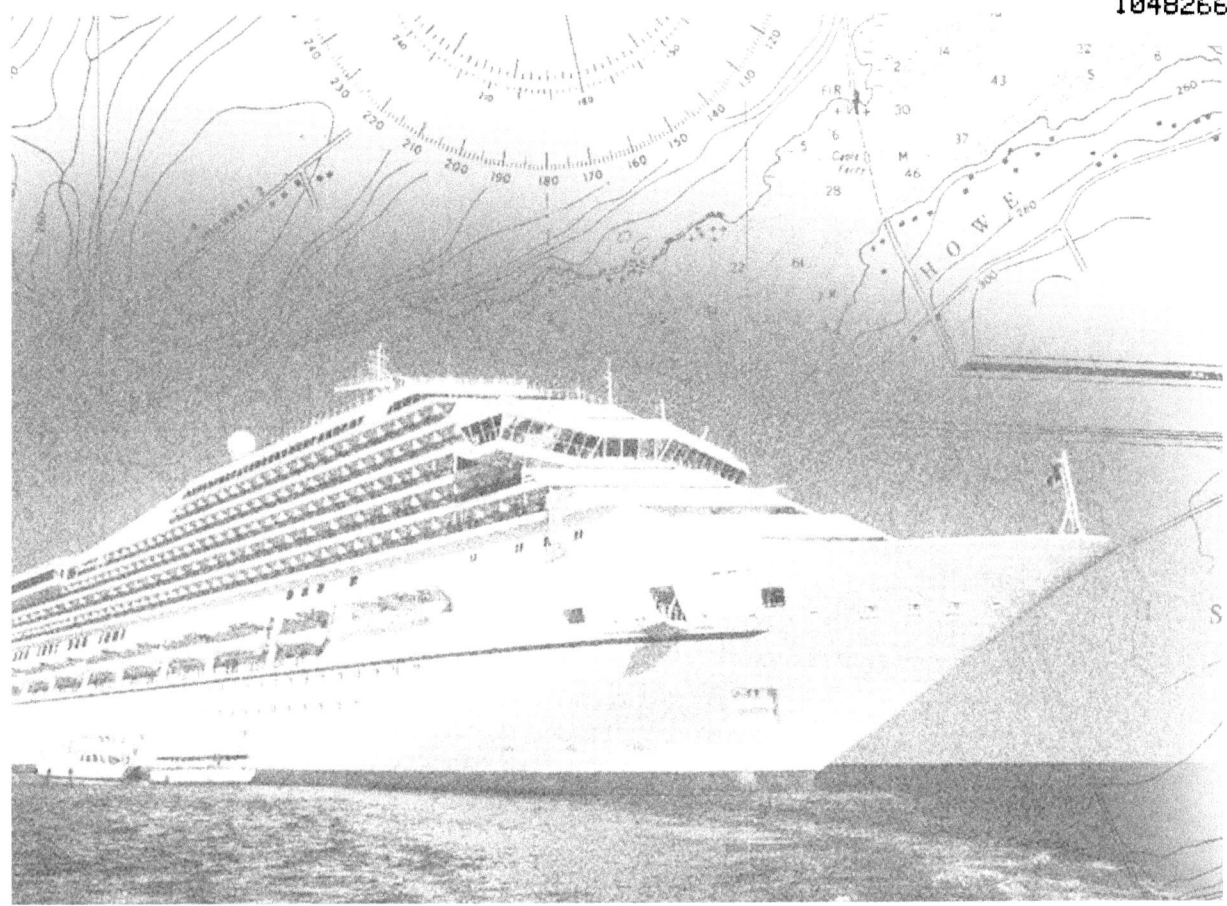

U.S. Department of Health and Human Services

U.S. Public Health Service

Centers for Disease Control and Prevention/
National Center for Environmental Health

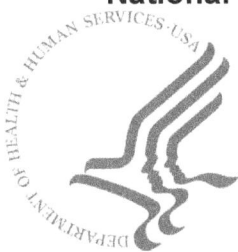
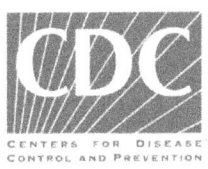
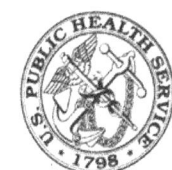

Vessel Sanitation Program
Centers for Disease Control and Prevention
4770 Buford Highway, NE/MS F-59
Atlanta, GA 30341-3717
Phone: 770-488-7070
Fax: 770-488-4127
E-mail: vsp@cdc.gov

Vessel Sanitation Program
Centers for Disease Control and Prevention
1850 Eller Drive, Suite 101
Ft. Lauderdale, FL 33316-4201
Phone: 800-323-2132 or 954-356-6650
Fax: 954-356-6671
E-mail: vsp@cdc.gov

The *VSP 2011 Construction Guidelines* and updates are available at
http://www.cdc.gov/nceh/vsp.

Acknowledgments

VSP would like to acknowledge the following organizations and companies for their cooperative efforts in the revisions of the *VSP 2011 Construction Guidelines*.

Cruise lines
- AIDA Cruises
- Carnival Corporation & PLC
- Carnival Cruise Line
- Carnival UK (P&O Cruises and Cunard)
- Disney Cruise Line
- Holland America Line
- Norwegian Cruise Line
- MSC Cruises
- Prestige Cruise Holdings (Oceania and Regent Seven Seas Cruises)
- Princess Cruises
- Royal Caribbean Cruises Ltd. (Royal Caribbean International, Celebrity Cruises, and Azamara Cruises)

Shipyards
- Fincantieri Cantieri Navali Italiani SpA
- Meyer Werft GmbH
- STX Europe (France and Finland)
- T. Mariotti SpA

Other Organizations
- ALMACO Group, SAS
- Bill Aleman, Inc.
- Culligan Italiana S.p.A.
- Cruise Lines International Association (CLIA)
- D$_2$ Marine Solutions, Inc.
- DL Forney Consulting
- DL SERVICES
- Ecolab
- EU SHIPSAN
- Health Canada
- HOBART Global Marine
- Italcatering (MSC Cruises)
- JP Schnoor Consulting
- MEIKO Maschinenbau GmbH & CO KG
- MEIKO USA
- MKN Gmbh & Co.
- O.T. S.r.l
- Precetti SpA
- Prescott Consulting
- SeaKing Ltd.
- TGMG, Inc.
- Tuttle Training Institute
- Walt Disney Imagineering
- World Health Organization

The cover art was designed by Carrie Green.

Contents

1.0 Background and Purpose

The Centers for Disease Control and Prevention (CDC) established the Vessel Sanitation Program (VSP) in 1975 as a cooperative endeavor with the cruise vessel industry. VSP's goal is to assist the industry to develop and implement comprehensive sanitation programs to protect the health of passengers and crew aboard cruise vessels.

Every cruise vessel that has a foreign itinerary, carries 13 or more passengers, and calls on a U.S. port is subject to biannual operational inspections and, when necessary, reinspection by VSP. The vessel owner pays a fee, based on gross registered tonnage (GRT) of the vessel, for all operational inspections. The *Vessel Sanitation Program 2011 Operations Manual*, which is available on the VSP Web site (www.cdc.gov/nceh/vsp), covers details of these inspections.

Additionally, cruise vessel owners or shipyards that build or renovate cruise vessels may voluntarily request plan reviews, onsite shipyard construction inspections, and/or final construction inspections of new or renovated vessels before their first or next operational inspection. The vessel owner or shipyard pays a fee, based on GRT of the vessel, for onsite and final construction inspections. VSP does not charge a fee for plan reviews or consultations. Section 3.0 covers details pertaining to plan reviews, consultations, or construction inspections.

When a plan review or construction inspection is requested, VSP reviews current construction billing invoices of the shipyard or owner requesting the inspection. If this review identifies construction invoices unpaid for more than 90 days, no inspection will be scheduled. An inspection can be scheduled after the outstanding invoices are paid in full.

These guidelines were published in 1997 and 2001 as the *Recommended Shipbuilding Construction Guidelines for Cruise Vessels Destined to Call on U.S. Ports*. In 2005, the guidelines were renamed as the *Vessel Sanitation Program 2005 Construction Guidelines*.

The *VSP 2011 Construction Guidelines* provide a framework of consistent construction and design guidelines that protect passenger and crew health. CDC is committed to promoting high construction standards to protect the public's health. Compliance with these guidelines will help to ensure a healthy environment on cruise vessels.

CDC reviewed references from many sources to develop these guidelines. These references are indicated in section 38.2.

The *VSP 2011 Construction Guidelines* cover components of the vessel's facilities related to public health, including FOOD STORAGE, PREPARATION, and SERVICE, and water bunkering, storage, DISINFECTION, and distribution. Vessel owners and operators may select the design and equipment that best meets their needs. However, the design and equipment must also meet the sanitary design criteria of the American National Standards Institute (ANSI) or equivalent organization as well as VSP's routine operational inspection requirements.

These guidelines are not meant to limit the introduction of new designs, materials, or technology for shipbuilding. A shipbuilder, owner, manufacturer, or other interested party may ask VSP to periodically review or revise these guidelines in relation to new information or technology. VSP reviews such requests in accordance with the criteria described in section 2.0.

New cruise vessels must comply with all international code requirements (e.g., International Maritime Organization Conventions). Those include requirements of the following:
- Safety of Life-at-Sea Convention.
- International Convention for the Prevention of Pollution from Ships.
- Tonnage and Load Line Convention.
- International Electrical Code.
- International Plumbing Code.
- International Standards Organization.

This document does not cross-reference related and sometimes overlapping standards that new cruise vessels must meet.

The *VSP 2011 Construction Guidelines* went into effect on September 15, 2011. They apply to vessels that LAY KEEL or perform any major renovation or equipment replacement (e.g., any changes to the structural elements of the vessel covered by these guidelines) after this date. The guidelines do not apply to minor renovations such as the installation or removal of single pieces of equipment (refrigerator units, warewash machines, bain-marie units, etc.) or single pipe runs. These guidelines apply to all areas of the vessel affected by a renovation. VSP will inspect the entire vessel in accordance with the *VSP 2011 Operations Manual* during routine vessel sanitation inspections and reinspections.

2.0   Revisions and Changes

VSP periodically reviews and revises these recommendations in coordination with industry representatives and other interested parties to stay abreast with industry innovations. A shipbuilder, owner, manufacturer, or other interested party may ask VSP to review a construction guideline on the basics of new technologies, concepts, or methods.

Recommendations for changes or additions to these guidelines must be submitted in writing to the VSP Chief (see section 39.2.1 for contact information). The recommendation should
- Identify the section to be revised.
- Describe the proposed change or addition.
- State the reason for recommending the change or addition.
- Include research or test results and any other pertinent information that support the change or addition.

VSP will coordinate a professional evaluation and consult with industry to determine whether to include the recommendation in the next revision.

VSP gives special consideration to shipyards and owners of vessels that have had plan reviews conducted before an effective date of a revision of these guidelines. This helps limit any burden placed on the shipyards and owners to make excessive changes to previously agreed-upon plans.

VSP asks industry representatives and other knowledgeable parties to meet with VSP representatives periodically to review the guidelines and determine whether changes are necessary to keep up with the innovations in the industry.

3.0 Procedures for Requesting Plan Reviews, Consultations, and Construction-related Inspections

To coordinate or schedule a plan review or construction-related inspection, submit an official written request to the VSP Chief as early as possible in the planning, construction, or renovation process. Requests that require foreign travel must be received in writing at least 45 days before the intended visit. The request will be honored depending on VSP staff availability (see section 39.2.1 for contact information).

After the initial contact, VSP assigns primary and secondary officers to coordinate with the vessel owner and shipyard. Normally two officers will be assigned. These officers are the points of contact for the vessel from the time the plan review and subsequent consultations take place through the final construction inspection.

Vessel representatives should provide points of contact to represent the owners, shipyard, and key subcontractors. All parties will use these points of contact during consultations between any of the parties and VSP to ensure awareness of all consultative activities after the plan review is conducted.

3.1 Plan Reviews and Consultations

VSP normally conducts plan reviews for new construction a minimum of 18 months before the vessel is scheduled for delivery. The time required for major renovations varies. To allow time for any necessary changes, VSP coordinates plan reviews for such projects well before the work begins.

Plan reviews normally take 2 working days. They are conducted in Atlanta, Georgia; Fort Lauderdale, Florida; or other agreed-upon sites. Normally, two VSP officers will be assigned to the project.

Representatives from the shipyard, vessel owner, and subcontractor(s) who will be doing most of the work should attend the review. They should bring all pertinent materials for areas covered in these guidelines, including (but not limited to) the following:
- Complete plans or drawings (this includes new vessels from a class built under a previous version of the *VSP Construction Guidelines*).
- Any available menus.
- Equipment specifications.
- General arrangement plans.

- Decorative materials for FOOD AREAS and bars.
- All FOOD-related STORAGE, PREPARATION, and SERVICE AREA plans.
- Level and type of FOOD SERVICE (e.g., concept menus, staffing plans, etc.).
- POTABLE and nonpotable water system plans with details on water inlets, (e.g., sea chests, overboard discharge points, and BACKFLOW PREVENTION DEVICES).
- Ventilation system plans.
- Plans for all RECREATIONAL WATER FACILITIES.
- Size profiles for operational areas.
- Owner-supplied and PORTABLE equipment specifications, including cleaning procedures.
- Cabin attendant work zones.
- Operational schematics for misting systems and decorative fountains.

VSP will prepare a plan review report summarizing recommendations made during the plan review and will submit the report to the shipyard and owner representatives.

Following the plan review, the shipyard will provide the following:
- Any redrawn plans.
- Copies of any major change orders made after the plan review in areas covered by these guidelines.

While the vessel is being built, shipyard representatives, the ship owner, or other vessel representatives may direct questions or requests for consultative services to the VSP project officers. Direct these questions or requests in writing to the officer(s) assigned to the project. Include fax number(s) and an e-mail address(es) for appropriate contacts. The VSP officer(s) will coordinate the request with the owner and shipyard points of contact designated during the plan review.

3.2   Onsite Construction Inspections

VSP conducts most onsite or shipyard construction inspections in shipyards outside the United States. A formal written request must be submitted to the VSP Chief at least 45 days before the inspection date so that VSP can process the required foreign travel orders for VSP officers (see section 3.0). A sample request is shown in section 39.1.

A completed vessel profile sheet must also be submitted with the request for the onsite inspection (see section 40.0). VSP encourages shipyards to contact the VSP Chief and coordinate onsite construction inspections well before the 45-day minimum to better plan the actual inspection dates. If a shipyard requests an onsite construction inspection, VSP will advise the vessel owner of the inspection dates so that the owner's representatives are present.

An onsite construction inspection normally requires the expertise of one to three officers, depending on the size of the vessel and whether it is the first of a hull design class or a subsequent hull in a series of the same class of vessels. The inspection, including travel, generally takes 5 working days. The onsite inspection should be conducted approximately 4 to 5 weeks before delivery of the vessel when 90% of the areas of the vessel to be inspected are completed. VSP will provide a written report to the party that requested the inspection. After the inspection and before the ship's arrival in the United States, the shipyard will submit to VSP a statement of corrective action outlining how it will address and correct each item identified in the inspection report.

3.3   Final Construction Inspections

3.3.1   Purpose and Scheduling

At the request of a vessel owner or shipyard, VSP may conduct a final construction inspection. Final construction inspections are conducted only after construction is 100% complete and the ship is fully operational.

These inspections are conducted to evaluate the findings of the previous yard inspection, assess all areas that were incomplete in the previous yard inspection, and evaluate performance tests on systems that could not be tested in the previous yard inspection. Such systems include the following:
- Ventilation for cooking, holding, and warewashing areas.
- Warewash machines.
- Artificial light levels.
- Temperatures in cold or hot holding equipment.
- HALOGEN and other chemistry measures for POTABLE WATER or RECREATIONAL WATER systems.

To schedule the inspection, the vessel owner or shipyard submits a formal written request to the VSP Chief as soon as possible after the vessel is completed, or a minimum of 10 days before its arrival in the United States. At the request of a vessel owner or shipyard and provided the vessel is not entering the U.S. market immediately, VSP may conduct final construction inspections outside the United States (see section 3.2 for foreign inspection procedures).

As soon as possible after the final construction inspection, the vessel owner or shipyard will submit a statement of corrective action to VSP. The statement outlines how the shipyard will address each item cited in the inspection report and includes the projected date of completion.

3.3.2   Unannounced Operational Inspection

VSP generally schedules vessels that undergo final construction inspection in the United States for an unannounced operational inspection within 4 weeks of the vessel's final construction inspection. VSP conducts operational inspections in accordance with the *VSP 2011 Operations Manual*.

If a final construction inspection is not requested, VSP generally will conduct an unannounced operational inspection within 4 weeks after the vessel's arrival in the United States. VSP conducts operational inspections in accordance with the *VSP 2011 Operations Manual.*

4.0   Equipment Standards, Testing, and Certification

Although these guidelines establish certain standards for equipment and materials installed on cruise vessels, VSP does not test, certify, or otherwise endorse or approve any equipment or materials used by the cruise industry. Instead, VSP recognizes certification from independent testing laboratories such as NSF International, Underwriter's Laboratories (UL), the American National Standards Institute (ANSI), and other recognized independent international testing institutions.

In most cases, independent testing laboratories test equipment and materials to certain minimum standards that generally meet the recommended standards established by these guidelines. Equipment built to questionable standards will be reviewed by a committee consisting of VSP, cruise ship industry, and independent testing organization participants. The committee will determine whether the equipment meets the recommended standards established in these guidelines. Copies of test or certification standards are available from the independent testing laboratories.

Equipment manufacturers and suppliers should not contact the VSP to request approval of their products.

5.0   General Definitions and Acronyms

5.1   Scope

These *VSP 2011 Construction Guidelines* provide definitions to clarify commonly used terminology in this manual. The definition section is organized alphabetically.

Terms defined in section 5.2 are identified in the text of these guidelines by SMALL CAPITAL LETTERS, or SMALL CAPS. For example: section 6.2.5 states "Provide READILY REMOVABLE DRIP TRAYS for condiment dispensing equipment." READILY REMOVABLE and DRIP TRAYS are in SMALL CAPS and are defined in section 5.2.

5.2   Definitions

Accessible: Exposed for cleaning and inspection with the use of simple tools such as a screwdriver, pliers, or wrench.

Activity pools: Include but are not limited to the following: wave pools, catch pools, water slides, INTERACTIVE RECREATIONAL WATER FACILITIES, lazy rivers, action rivers, vortex pools, and continuous surface pools.

Adequate: Sufficient in number, features, or capacity to accomplish the purpose for which something is intended and to such a degree that there is no unreasonable risk to health or safety.

Air-break: A piping arrangement in which a drain from a fixture, appliance, or device discharges indirectly into another fixture, receptacle, or interceptor at a point below the flood-level rim (Figure 1).

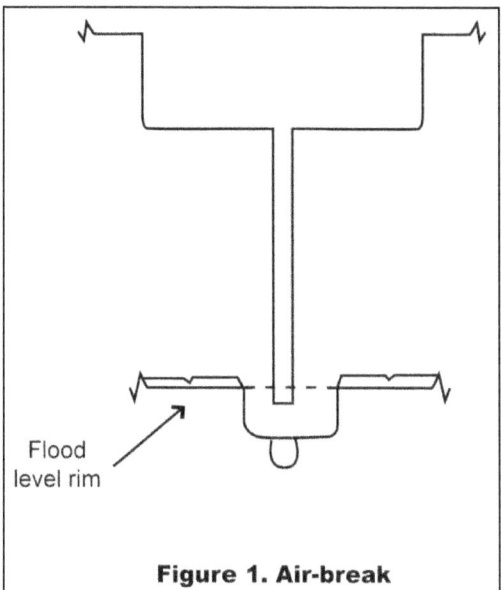

Flood
level rim

Figure 1. Air-break

Air gap: (AG) The unobstructed vertical distance through the free atmosphere between the lowest opening from any pipe or faucet supplying water to a tank, PLUMBING FIXTURE, or other device and the flood-level rim of the receptacle or receiving fixture. The air gap must be at least twice the inside diameter of the supply pipe or faucet and not less than 25 millimeters (1 inch) (Figure 2). Manufactured air gaps must be certified by a recognized plumbing or engineering organization.

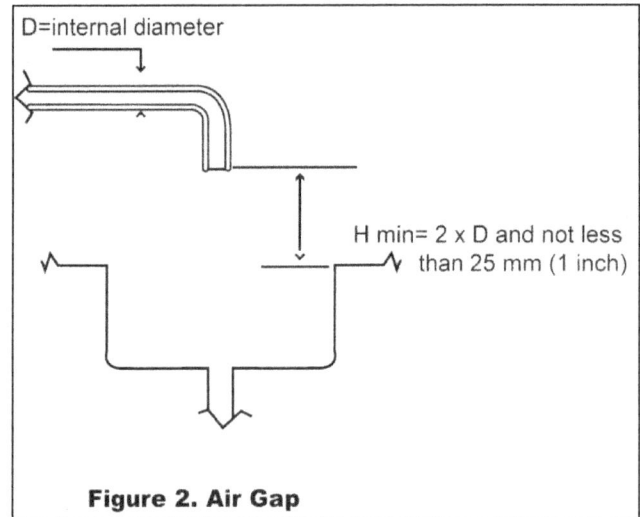

Figure 2. Air Gap

Antientanglement cover: A cover for a BLOCKABLE DRAIN/SUCTION FITTING that is designed to prevent hair from tangling in a BLOCKABLE DRAIN cover or SUCTION FITTING in a RECREATIONAL WATER FACILITY.

Antientrapment cover: A cover for a BLOCKABLE DRAIN/SUCTION FITTING that is designed to prevent any portion of the body or hair from becoming lodged or otherwise forced onto a BLOCKABLE DRAIN cover or SUCTION FITTING in a RECREATIONAL WATER FACILITY.

Approved: Acceptable based on a determination of conformity with principles, practices, and generally recognized standards that protect public health (e.g., American National Standards Institute [ANSI], National Sanitation Foundation International [NSF International], American Society of Mechanical Engineers [ASME], or American Society of Safety Engineers [ASSE] standards, Underwriter's Laboratories [UL], federal regulations, or equivalent international standards and regulations).

Atmospheric vacuum breaker (AVB): A BACKFLOW PREVENTION DEVICE that consists of an air inlet valve, a check seat or float valve, and air inlet ports. The device is not APPROVED for use under continuous water pressure and must be installed downstream of the last valve.

Automatic pump shut-off (APS): System device that can sense a BLOCKABLE DRAIN blockage and shut off the pumps in a RECREATIONAL WATER FACILITY.

Baby-only water facility: RECREATIONAL WATER FACILITY designed for use by children in diapers or children who are not completely toilet trained. This facility must have zero water depth. Control measures for this facility would be detailed in a variance. For the operation of this facility, a variance would be required.

Backflow: The reversal of flow of water or other liquids, mixtures, or substances into the distribution pipes of a POTABLE supply of water from any source or sources other than the source of POTABLE WATER supply. BACKSIPHONAGE and BACKPRESSURE are forms of backflow.

Backflow prevention device: An APPROVED plumbing device that must be used on POTABLE WATER distribution lines where there is a direct connection or a potential CROSS-CONNECTION between the POTABLE WATER distribution system and other liquids, mixtures, or substances from any source other than the POTABLE WATER supply. Some devices are designed for use under continuous water pressure, whereas others are noncontinuous pressure types. VSP only accepts vented devices.

(See also:
- ATMOSPHERIC VACUUM BREAKER.
- CONTINUOUS PRESSURE BACKFLOW PREVENTION DEVICE.
- DOUBLE CHECK VALVE WITH INTERMEDIATE ATMOSPHERIC VENT.
- HOSE BIB CONNECTION VACUUM BREAKER.
- PRESSURE VACUUM BREAKER ASSEMBLY.
- REDUCED PRESSURE PRINCIPLE BACKFLOW PREVENTION ASSEMBLY).

Backpressure: An elevation of pressure in the downstream piping system (by pump, elevation of piping, or steam and/or air pressure) above the supply pressure at the point of consideration that would cause a reversal of normal direction of flow.

Backsiphonage: The reversal of flow of used, contaminated, or polluted water from a PLUMBING FIXTURE or vessel or other source into a water supply pipe as a result of negative pressure in the pipe.

Black water: Wastewater from toilets, urinals, medical sinks, and other similar facilities.

Blast chiller: A unit specifically designed for rapid cooling of food products.

Blockable drain/suction fitting: A drain or suction fitting in a RECREATIONAL WATER FACILITY that that can be completely covered or blocked by a 457 millimeters x 584 millimeters (18 inches x 23 inches) body-blocking element as set forth in ASME A112.19.8M.

Child activity center: A facility for child-related activities where children under the age of 6 are placed to be cared for by vessel staff.

Children's pool: A pool that has a depth of 1 meter (3 feet) or less and is intended for use by children who are toilet trained.

Child-sized toilet: Toilets whose toilet seat height is no more than 280 millimeters (11 inches) and the toilet seat opening is no greater than 203 millimeters (8 inches).

Cleaning locker: A room or cabinet specifically designed or modified for storage of cleaning equipment such as mops, brooms, floor-scrubbing machines, and cleaning chemicals.

Continuous pressure (CP) backflow prevention device: A device generally consisting of two check valves and an intermediate atmospheric vent that has been specifically designed to be used under conditions of continuous pressure (greater than 12 hours out of a 24-hour period).

Coved (also coving): A curved or concave surface, molding, or other design that eliminates the usual joint angles of 90° or less. A single piece of stainless steel bent to an angle not less than 90° with a minimum 9.5-millimeter radius is acceptable (Figures 3-5). Unique circumstances for coving can be reviewed during plan review.

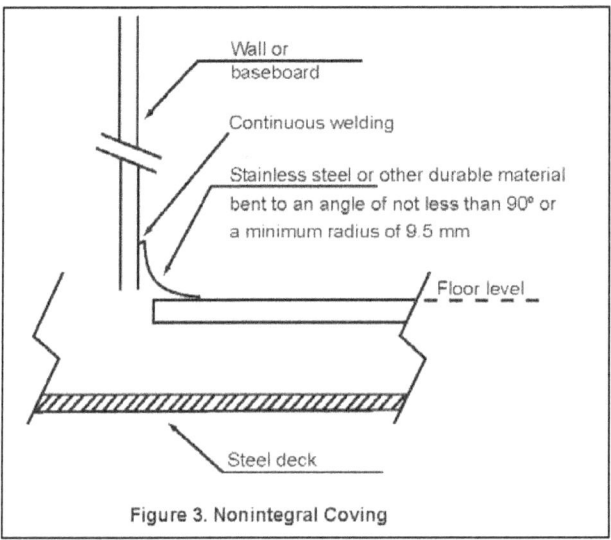

Figure 3. Nonintegral Coving

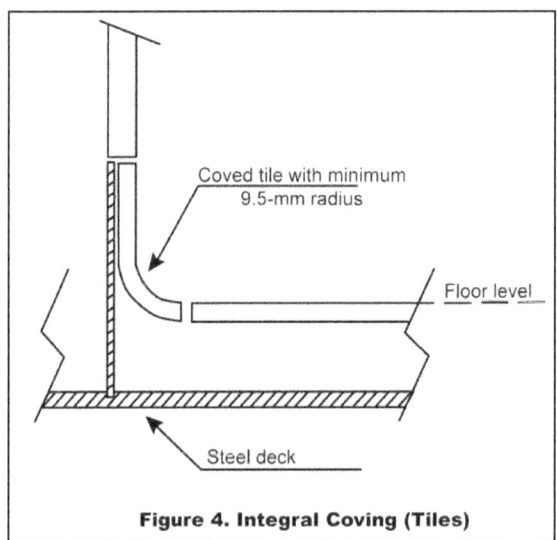

Figure 4. Integral Coving (Tiles)

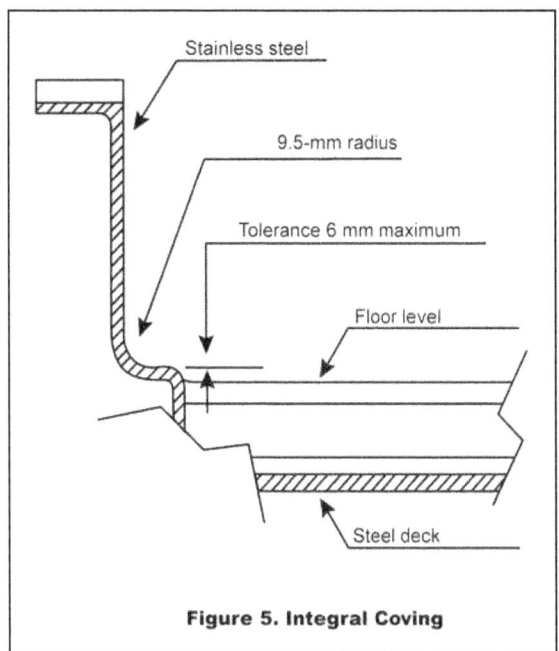

Figure 5. Integral Coving

Cross-connection: An actual or potential connection or structural arrangement between a POTABLE WATER system and any other source or system through which it is possible to introduce into any part of the POTABLE WATER system any used water, industrial fluid, gas, or substance other than the intended POTABLE WATER with which the system is supplied.

Deck drain: The physical connection between decks, SCUPPERS, or DECK SINKS and the GRAY or BLACK WATER systems.

Deck sink: A sink recessed into the deck and sized to contain waste liquids from tilting kettles and pans.

Disinfection: A process (physical or chemical) that destroys many or all pathogenic microorganisms, except bacterial and mycotic spores, on inanimate objects.

Distillate water lines: Pipes carrying water that is condensed from the evaporators and that may be directed to the POTABLE WATER system. This is the VSP definition for pipe striping purposes.

Double check (DC) valve assembly: A BACKFLOW PREVENTION ASSEMBLY consisting of two internally loaded, independently operating check valves that are located between two resilient-seated shut-off valves. These assemblies include four resilient-seated test cocks. **These devices do not have an intermediate vent to the atmosphere and are not APPROVED for use on CROSS-CONNECTIONS to the POTABLE WATER system of cruise vessels. VSP accepts only vented BACKFLOW PREVENTION DEVICES.**

Double check with intermediate atmospheric vent (DCIV): A BACKFLOW PREVENTION DEVICE with double check valves and an intermediate atmospheric vent located between the two check valves.

Drip tray: READILY REMOVABLE tray to collect dripping fluids or food from food dispensing equipment.

Dry storage area: A room or area designated for the storage of packaged or containerized bulk food that is not potentially hazardous and dry goods such as single-service items.

Dual swing check valve: A nonreturn device installed on RECREATIONAL WATER FACILITY drain pipes when connected to another drainage system. This device is not APPROVED for use on the POTABLE WATER system.

Easily cleanable: A characteristic of a surface that
- Allows effective removal of soil by normal cleaning methods;
- Is dependent on the material, design, construction, and installation of the surface; and
- Varies with the likelihood of the surface's role in introducing pathogenic or toxigenic agents or other contaminants into food based on the surface's APPROVED placement, purpose, and use.

Easily movable: Equipment that
- Is PORTABLE; mounted on casters, gliders, or rollers; or provided with a mechanical means to safely tilt it for cleaning; and
- Has no utility connection, has a utility connection that disconnects quickly, or has a flexible utility connection line of sufficient length that allows it to be moved for cleaning of the equipment and adjacent area.

Food area: Includes food and beverage DISPLAY, HANDLING, PREPARATION, SERVICE, and STORAGE AREAS; warewash areas; clean equipment storage areas; and table linen storage and handling areas.

Food-contact surface: Surfaces (food zone, splash zone) of equipment and utensils with which food normally comes in contact and surfaces from which food may drain, drip, or splash back into a food or surfaces normally in contact with food (Figure 6).

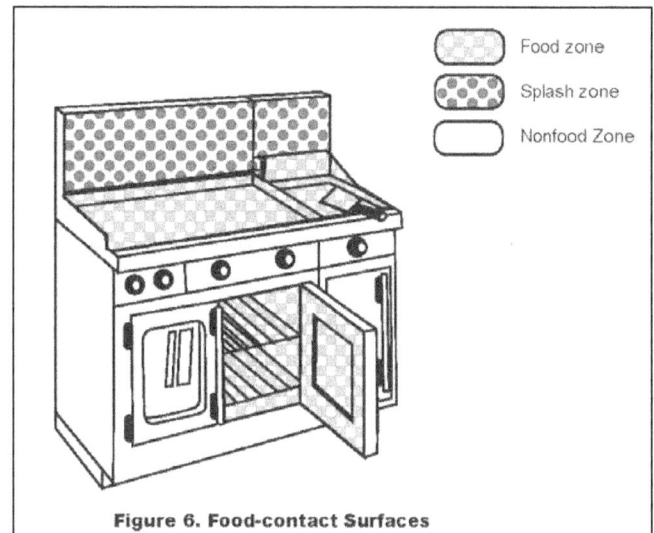

Figure 6. Food-contact Surfaces

Food display areas: Any area where food is displayed for consumption by passengers and/or crew. Applies to displays served by vessel staff or self service.

Food-handling areas: Any area where food is stored, processed, prepared, or served.

Food preparation areas: Any area where food is processed, cooked, or prepared for service.

Food service areas: Any area where food is presented to passengers or crew members (excluding individual cabin service).

Food storage areas: Any area where food or food products are stored.

Food transportation corridors: Areas primarily intended to move food during FOOD PREPARATION, STORAGE, and SERVICE operations (e.g., service lift [elevator] vestibules to FOOD PREPARATION SERVICE and STORAGE AREAS, provision corridors, and corridors connecting preparation areas and service areas). **Passenger and crew corridors, public areas, individual cabin service, and dining rooms connected to galleys are excluded. Food loading areas used solely for delivery of food to the vessel are excluded. Corridors within a galley are to be constructed to galley standards.**

Food waste system: A system used to collect, transport, and process food waste from FOOD AREAS to a waste disposal system (e.g., pulper, vacuum system).

Gap: An open juncture that is more than 3 millimeters (1/8 inch).

Gravity drain: A drain fitting used to drain the body of water in a RECREATIONAL WATER FACILITY by gravity and with no pump downstream of the fitting.

Gravity drainage system: A water collection system whereby a collection tank is located between the RECREATIONAL WATER FACILITY and the suction pumps.

Gray water: Wastewater from galley equipment and DECK DRAINS, dishwashers, showers and baths, laundries, washbasins, DECK DRAINS, and recirculated RECREATIONAL WATER FACILITIES. Gray water does not include BLACK WATER or bilge water from the machinery spaces.

Gutterway: See SCUPPER.

Halogen: The group of elements including chlorine, bromine, and iodine used for the DISINFECTION of water.

Hose bib connection vacuum breaker (HVB): A BACKFLOW PREVENTION DEVICE that attaches directly to a hose bib by way of a threaded head. This device uses a single check valve and vacuum breaker vent. It is not APPROVED for use under CONTINUOUS PRESSURE (e.g., when a shut-off valve is located downstream from the device). This device is a form of an AVB specifically designed for a hose connection.

Interactive recreational water facilities: Structures that provide a variety of recreational water features such as flowing, misting, sprinkling, jetting, and waterfalls. These facilities may be zero depth.

Keel laying: The date at which construction identifiable with a specific ship begins and when assembly of that ship comprises at least 50 tons or 1% of the estimated mass of all structural material, whichever is less.

mg/L: Milligrams per liter, the metric equivalent of parts per million (ppm).

Noncorroding: Material that maintains its original surface characteristics through prolonged influence by the use environment, food contact, and normal use of cleaning compounds and sanitizing solutions.

Nonfood-contact surfaces (nonfood zone): All exposed surfaces, other than FOOD-CONTACT SURFACES, of equipment located in FOOD AREAS (Figure 6).

Permeate water lines: Pipes carrying permeate water from the reverse osmosis unit that may be directed to the POTABLE WATER system. This is the VSP definition for pipe striping purposes.

pH (Potens hydrogen): The symbol for the negative logarithm of the hydrogen ion concentration, which is a measure of the degree of acidity or alkalinity of a solution. Values between 0 and 7 indicate acidity and values between 7 and 14 indicate alkalinity. The value for pure distilled water is 7, which is neutral.

Plumbing fixture: A receptacle or device that
- Is permanently or temporarily connected to the water-distribution system of the vessel and demands a supply of water from the system; or
- Discharges used water, waste materials, or SEWAGE directly or indirectly to the drainage system of the vessel.

Portable: A description of equipment that is READILY REMOVABLE or mounted on casters, gliders, or rollers; provided with a mechanical means so that it can be tilted safely for cleaning; or EASILY MOVABLE by one person.

Potable water: Water that is HALOGENATED and pH controlled and is intended for
- drinking, washing, bathing, or showering;
- use in fresh water SWIMMING POOLS and WHIRLPOOL SPAS;
- use in the vessel's hospital;
- handling, preparing, or cooking food; and
- cleaning FOOD STORAGE and PREPARATION areas, utensils, and equipment.

Potable water is free from impurities in amounts sufficient to cause disease or harmful physiological effects. The water quality must conform to requirements of the World Health Organization drinking water standards.

Potable water tanks: All tanks in which potable water is stored for use in the POTABLE WATER system.

Pressure vacuum breaker assembly (PVB): A device consisting of an independently loaded internal check valve and a spring-loaded air inlet valve. This device is also equipped with two resilient seated gate valves and test cocks.

Readily accessible: Exposed or capable of being exposed for cleaning or inspection without the use of tools.

Readily removable: Capable of being detached from the main unit without the use of tools.

Recreational seawater: Seawater taken onboard while making way at a position at least 12 miles at sea and routed directly to the RWFs for either sea-to-sea exchange or recirculation.

Recreational water facility (RWF): A water facility that has been modified, improved, constructed, or installed for the purpose of public swimming or recreational bathing. RWFs include, but are not limited to,
- ACTIVITY POOLS.
- BABY-ONLY WATER FACILITIES.
- CHILDREN'S POOLS.
- Diving pools.
- Hot tubs.

- Hydrotherapy pools.
- INTERACTIVE RECREATIONAL WATER FACILITIES.
- Slides.
- SPA POOLS.
- SWIMMING POOLS.
- Therapeutic pools.
- WADING POOLS.
- WHIRLPOOLS.

Reduced pressure principle backflow prevention assembly (RP assembly): An assembly containing two independently acting internally loaded check valves together with a hydraulically operating, mechanically independent pressure differential relief valve located between the check valves and at the same time below the first check valve. The unit must include properly located resilient seated test cocks and tightly closing resilient seated shutoff valves at each end of the assembly.

Removable: Capable of being detached from the main unit with the use of simple tools such as a screwdriver, pliers, or an open-end wrench.

Safety vacuum release system (SVRS): A system that is capable of releasing a vacuum at a suction outlet caused by a high vacuum due to a blockage in the outlet flow. These systems shall be designed and certified in accordance with ASTM F2387-04 or ANSI/ASME A 112.19.17-2002.

Sanitary seawater lines: Water lines with seawater intended for use in the POTABLE WATER production systems or in RECREATIONAL WATER FACILITIES.

Scupper: A conduit or collection basin that channels liquid runoff to a DECK DRAIN.

Sealant: Material used to fill SEAMS.

Seam: An open juncture that is greater than 0.8 millimeters (1/32 inch) but less than 3 millimeters (1/8 inch).

Smooth:
- A FOOD-CONTACT SURFACE having a surface free of pits and inclusions with a cleanability equal to or exceeding that of (100-grit) number 3 stainless steel.
- A NONFOOD-CONTACT SURFACE of equipment having a surface equal to that of commercial grade hot-rolled steel free of visible scale.
- Deck, bulkhead, or deckhead that has an even or level surface with no roughness or projections to make it difficult to clean.

Spa pool: A POTABLE WATER or saltwater-supplied pool with temperatures and turbulence comparable to a WHIRLPOOL SPA.

General characteristics are
- Water temperature of 30°C-40°C or 86°F-104°F.
- Bubbling, jetted, or sprayed water effects that physically break at or above the water surface.
- Depth of more than 1 meter (3 feet).
- Tub volume of more than 6 tons of water.

Spill-resistant vacuum breaker (SVB): A specific modification to a PVB to minimize water spillage.

Spray pad: The play and water contact area that is designed to have no standing water.

Suction fitting: A fitting in a RECREATIONAL WATER FACILITY under direct suction through which water is drawn by a pump.

Swimming pool: A RECREATIONAL WATER FACILITY greater than 1 meter in depth. This does not include SPA POOLS that meet this depth.

Technical water: Water that has not been chlorinated or PH controlled and that originates from a bunkering or condensate collection process, or seawater processed through the evaporators or reverse osmosis plant and is intended for storage and use in the technical water system.

Temperature-measuring devices (TMDs): Thermometers, thermocouples, thermistors, or other devices that indicate the temperature of food, air, or water and are numerically scaled in Celsius and/or Fahrenheit. TMDs must be designed to be easily readable.

Turnover: The circulation, through the recirculation system, of a quantity of water equal to the total RWF tub volume. For facilities with zero depth, the turnover will be based on the total volume of the system, including compensation or make-up tanks and piping, and up to the entire volume for the system as designed.

Unblockable drain/suction fitting: A drain or suction fitting in a RECREATIONAL WATER FACILITY that cannot be completely covered or blocked by a 457 millimeters x 584 millimeters (18 inches x 23 inches) body-blocking element and that is rated by the test procedures or by the appropriate calculation in accordance with ASME A112.19.8M.

Utility sink: Any sink located in a FOOD SERVICE AREA not intended for handwashing and/or warewashing.

Wading pool: RECREATIONAL WATER FACILITY with a maximum depth of less than 1 meter and that is not designed for use by children.

Whirlpool spa: A freshwater or seawater pool designed to operate at a minimum temperature of 30°C (86°F) and maximum of 40°C (104°F) and equipped with either water or air jets. See also SPA POOL definition.

5.3 Acronyms

AG	AIR GAP
ANSI	American National Standards Institute
ASHRAE	American Society of Heating, Refrigeration and Air-Conditioning Engineers
ASME	American Society of Mechanical Engineers
ASSE	American Society of Safety Engineers
ASTM	American Society for Testing and Materials
AVB	ATMOSPHERIC VACUUM BREAKER
C	Celsius
CDC	Centers for Disease Control and Prevention
CP	continuous pressure
F	Fahrenheit
FDA	U.S. Food and Drug Administration
GRT	gross registered tonnage
HVB	HOSE-BIB CONNECTED VACUUM BREAKER
IEC	International Electrical Code
IMO	International Maritime Organization
IPC	International Plumbing Code
ISO	International Standards Organization
MARPOL	International Convention for the Prevention of Pollution from Ships
MG/L	MILLIGRAMS PER LITER
NCEH	National Center for Environmental Health
NSF International	National Sanitation Foundation International
ORP	oxidation reduction potential
pH	POTENS HYDROGEN
PHS	U.S. Public Health Service (also USPHS)
ppm	parts per million
RP ASSEMBLY	REDUCED PRESSURE PRINCIPLE BACKFLOW PREVENTION ASSEMBLY
RWF	RECREATIONAL WATER FACILITY
SOLAS	safety of life-at-sea
UL	Underwriter's Laboratories
UV	ultraviolet light
VSP	Vessel Sanitation Program
WHO	World Health Organization

6.0   General Facilities Requirements

6.1   Size and Flow

Many factors determine and influence the size of rooms and work areas and the flow of food through a vessel. Those factors can include the vessel size, number of passengers and crew, types of foods and menus, number of meals and mealtimes, service or presentation of meals, itinerary, and vessel owner's experience.

In general, FOOD STORAGE, PREPARATION, SERVICE and TRANSPORTATION areas; warewashing areas; and waste management areas must be sized to accommodate the vessel's full capacity of passengers and crew. Bulk FOOD STORAGE AREAS or provision rooms (e.g., frozen stores, refrigerated stores, and DRY STORAGE AREAS) must be sized to prevent the storage of bulk foods in provisions passageways unless the passageways are specifically designed to meet provision room standards (section 15.0). Refrigeration and hot-food holding facilities, including temporary storage facilities, must be available for all FOOD PREPARATION and SERVICE areas and for foods being transported to remote areas.

6.1.1   Food Flow

Arrange the flow of food through a vessel in a logical sequence that eliminates or minimizes cross-traffic or backtracking.

Provide a clear separation of clean and soiled operations. When a common corridor is used for movement of both clean and soiled operations, the minimum distance from bulkhead to bulkhead must be considered. Within a galley, the standard separation between clean and soiled operations must be a minimum of 2 meters (6½ feet). For smaller galleys (e.g., specialty, bell box) the minimum distance will be assessed during the plan review. Additionally, common corridors for size and flow of galley operations will be reviewed during the plan review.

Provide an orderly flow of food from the suppliers at dockside through the FOOD STORAGE, PREPARATION, and finishing areas to the SERVICE areas and, finally, to the waste management area. The goals are to reduce the risk for cross-contamination, prepare and serve food rapidly in accordance with strict time and temperature-control requirements, and minimize handling.

Provide a size profile for each FOOD AREA, including provisions, preparation rooms, galleys, pantries, warewash, garbage processing area, and storage. The size profile shows the square meters of space designated for that area. Where possible, the VSP will visit the profile vessel(s) to verify the capacity during operational inspections. The size profile must be an established standard for each cruise line based on the line's review of the area size for the same FOOD AREA in its existing vessels. As the ship size and passenger and crew totals change, there must be a proportional change in each FOOD AREA size based on the profile to ensure the service needs are met for each area. Size evaluations of FOOD AREAS will incorporate seating capacity and staffing, service, and equipment needs.

During the plan review process VSP evaluates the size of a particular room or area and the flow of food through the vessel to those rooms or areas. VSP will also use the results of operational inspections to review the size profiles submitted by individual cruise lines.

6.2   Equipment Requirements

6.2.1   Galleys

The equipment in sections 6.2.1.1 through 6.2.1.12 is required in galleys, depending on the level and type of service, and may be recommended for other areas.

6.2.1.1   *Blast Chillers*

Incorporate BLAST CHILLERS into the design of passenger and crew galleys. More than one unit may be necessary depending on the size of the vessel, and the distances between the BLAST CHILLERS and the storage and service areas.

6.2.1.1.1: The size and type of BLAST CHILLERS installed for each FOOD PREPARATION AREA are based on the concept/menu, operational requirements to satisfy that menu, and volume of food requiring cooling.

6.2.1.2   *Utility Sinks*

Include food preparation UTILITY SINKS in all meat, fish, and vegetable preparation rooms; in cold pantries or garde mangers; and in any other areas where personnel wash or soak food.

6.2.1.2.1: An automatic vegetable washing machine may be used in addition to FOOD PREPARATION UTILITY SINKS in vegetable preparation rooms.

6.2.1.3   *Food Storage*

Include storage cabinets, shelves, or racks for food products and equipment in FOOD STORAGE, PREPARATION, and SERVICE AREAS, including bars and pantries.

6.2.1.4   *Tables, Carts, or Pallets*

Locate fixed or PORTABLE tables, carts, or pallets in areas where food or ice is dispensed from cooking equipment, such as from soup kettles, steamers, braising pans, tilting pans, or ice storage bins.

6.2.1.5 Storage for Large Utensils

Include a storage cabinet or rack for large utensils such as ladles, paddles, whisks, and spatulas and provide for vertical storage of cutting boards.

6.2.1.6 Knife Storage

Include knife lockers or other designated knife storage facilities (e.g., drawers) that are EASILY CLEANABLE and meet food-contact standards.

6.2.1.7 Waiter Trays

Include storage areas, cabinets, or shelves for waiter trays.

6.2.1.8 Dish Storage

Include dishware lowerators or similar dish storage and dispensing cabinets.

6.2.1.9 Glass Rack

Include glass rack storage shelving.

6.2.1.10 Preparation Counters

Include work counters or food preparation counters that provide sufficient work space.

6.2.1.11 Drinking Fountains

Include drinking fountains that allow for hands-free operation and without a filling spout in FOOD AREAS.

6.2.1.12 Cleaning Lockers

Include CLEANING LOCKERS (see section 20.1 for specific CLEANING LOCKER construction requirements).

6.2.2 Warewashing Sinks

Equip the main galley, crew galley, and lido service area/galley pot washing areas with a three-compartment sink and prewash station or a four-compartment sink with an insert pan and an overhead spray.

Install sinks with compartments large enough to accommodate the largest piece of equipment (pots, tableware, etc.) used in their designated serving areas. An automatic warewash machine may be added but cannot be substituted for a three- or four-compartment sink.

Provide additional three-compartment sinks with prewash stations or four-compartment sinks with insert pans and overhead spray in heavy-use areas. These areas may include pastry/bakery, butcher shop, buffet pantry, and other preparation areas where the size of the facility or the location makes the use of a central pot washing area impractical.

6.2.3 Warewashing Access

Equip all FOOD PREPARATION AREAS with easy access to a three-compartment sink or a warewashing machine with an adjacent dump sink and prewash hose.

6.2.4 Drip Trays or Drains, Beverages

Furnish beverage dispensing equipment with READILY REMOVABLE DRIP TRAYS or built-in drains in the tabletop. Furnish bulk milk dispensers with READILY REMOVABLE DRIP TRAYS.

6.2.5 Drip Trays, Condiments

Provide READILY REMOVABLE DRIP TRAYS for condiment-dispensing equipment.

6.2.6 Equipment Storage Areas

Design storage areas to accommodate all equipment and utensils used in FOOD PREPARATION AREAS such as ladles and cutting blades.

6.2.7 Deck Drainage

Ensure that the design of installed equipment directs food and wash water drainage into a DECK DRAIN, SCUPPER, or DECK SINK, and not onto a deck.

6.2.8 Utility Sink

Provide a UTILITY SINK in areas such as beverage stations and bars where it is necessary to refill serving pitchers or discard beverages.

6.2.9 Dipper Wells

For hand-scooped ice cream, sherbet, or similar products, provide dipper wells with running water and proper drainage.

6.2.10 Doors or Closures

Provide tight-fitting doors or other protective closures for ice bins, FOOD DISPLAY cases, and other food and ice holding units to prevent contamination of stored products.

6.2.11 Countertop Openings and Rims

Protect countertop openings and rims of food cold tops, bains-marie, ice wells, and other drop-in type food and ice holding units with a raised integral edge (marine edge) or rim of at least 5 millimeters (3/16 inch) above the counter level around the opening.

6.3 Equipment Surfaces

6.3.1 Materials

Ensure that material used for FOOD-CONTACT SURFACES and exposed NONFOOD-CONTACT SURFACES are SMOOTH, durable, and NONCORRODING. They must be EASILY CLEANABLE and designed without unnecessary edges, projections, or crevices.

6.3.2 Approved Materials

Use only materials APPROVED for contact with food on FOOD-CONTACT SURFACES.

6.3.2.1 Surfaces

Make all FOOD-CONTACT SURFACES SMOOTH (with no sharp edges), durable, NONCORRODING, EASILY CLEANABLE, READILY ACCESSIBLE, and maintainable.

6.3.2.2 Corners

Provide COVED and seamless corners. Form external corners and angles with a sufficient radius to permit proper drainage and without sharp edges.

6.3.2.3 Sealants

Use only SEALANTS APPROVED for FOOD-CONTACT SURFACES (certified to ANSI/NSF Standard 51, or equivalent criteria) on FOOD-CONTACT SURFACES and food splash zone surfaces. Avoid excessive use of SEALANT.

6.3.3 Nonfood-contact Surfaces

Use durable and NONCORRODING material for NONFOOD-CONTACT SURFACES.

6.3.3.1 Easily Cleanable

Design NONFOOD-CONTACT SURFACES so that they are SMOOTH and EASILY CLEANABLE. Ensure that NONFOOD-CONTACT SURFACES are ACCESSIBLE for cleaning and maintenance.

6.3.3.2 No Sharp Corners

Ensure that NONFOOD-CONTACT SURFACES subject to food or beverage spills have no sharp internal corners and angles. Examples of these areas are waiter station work surfaces, beverage stations, technical compartments with drain lines, mess room soiled drop-off stations, and bus stations.

6.3.3.3 Compatible Metals

Use compatible metals to minimize corrosion due to galvanic action or provide effective insulation between dissimilar metals to protect them from corrosion.

6.4 Bulkheads, Deckheads, and Decks

6.4.1 Exposed Fasteners

Do not use exposed fasteners in bulkhead and deckhead construction.

6.4.2 Seams and Penetrations

Seal all SEAMS between adjoining bulkhead panels and adjoining deckhead panels and between bulkhead and deckhead panels.

6.4.2.1 Seal Seams

Seal SEAMS greater than 0.8 millimeters (1/32 inch), but less than 3 millimeters (1/8 inch), with an appropriate SEALANT or appropriate profile strips.

6.4.2.2 Cover Gaps

Cover all GAPS greater than 3 millimeters (1/8 inch) with appropriate profile strips.

6.4.2.3 Seal Penetrations

Seal all bulkhead, deckhead, and deck penetrations through which pipes or other conduits pass, including those located inside technical compartments. Use durable and NONCORRODING collars where GAPS are greater than 3 millimeters (1/8 inch).

6.4.3 Bulkheads

Reinforce all bulkheads sufficiently to prevent buckling or to prevent the bulkhead from becoming detached under normal operating conditions.

6.4.4 Door Penetrations

Weld door penetrations so that there are no exposed voids. Ensure that locking/latch pins insert into closed locking pin recesses. This also applies to the penetrations around fire doors, in thresholds, and in bulkhead openings. See Figure 7.

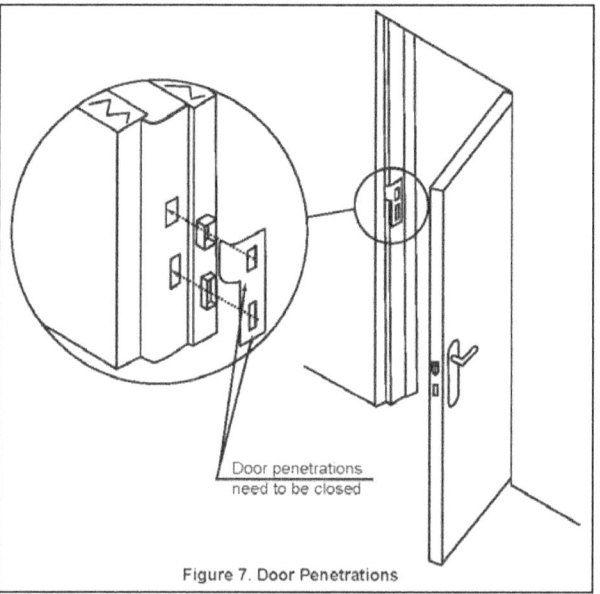

Door penetrations need to be closed

Figure 7. Door Penetrations

6.4.5 Deck Coving

Install COVING as an integral part of the deck and bulkhead interface and at the juncture between decks and equipment foundations.

6.4.5.1 Radius

Ensure COVING has at least a 9.5-millimeter (3/8 inch) radius or open design (> 90 degrees). Additionally, a single bent piece of stainless steel can be used as COVING. See COVING definition (Figures 3 and 4).

6.4.5.2 Materials

Provide COVING that is hard, durable, EASILY CLEANABLE, and of sufficient thickness to withstand normal wear.

6.4.5.3 Fasten

Securely fasten COVING.

6.4.6 Deck Material

Use material for decks that is hard, durable, EASILY CLEANABLE, nonskid, and nonabsorbent. Vinyl or linoleum deck coverings are not acceptable in FOOD AREAS. However, vinyl or linoleum deck coverings may be used in areas where only table linens are stored.

6.4.7 Compatible Metals

Use compatible metals to minimize corrosion due to galvanic action or provide effective insulation between dissimilar metals to protect them from corrosion.

6.5 Deck Drains, Deck Sinks, and Scuppers

6.5.1 Material

Construct DECK DRAINS, SCUPPERS, and DECK SINKS from stainless steel.

6.5.1.1 Other Requirements

Ensure DECK DRAINS, SCUPPERS, and DECK SINKS have SMOOTH finished surfaces, are ACCESSIBLE for cleaning, and are designed to drain completely.

6.5.2 Cover Grates

Construct SCUPPER, and DECK SINK cover grates from stainless steel or other materials that
- Meet the requirements for a SMOOTH, EASILY CLEANABLE surface,
- Are strong enough to maintain the original shape, and
- Have no sharp edges.

6.5.2.1 Other Requirements

Provide SCUPPER and DECK SINK cover grates that are tight-fitting, READILY REMOVABLE for cleaning, and uniform in length where practical (e.g., 1 meter or 40 inches) so that they are interchangeable.

6.5.3 Location

Place DECK DRAINS and DECK SINKS in low-traffic areas such as in front of soup kettles, boilers, tilting pans, or braising pans.

6.5.4   Sizing

Size DECK DRAINS, SCUPPERS, and sinks to eliminate spillage and overflow to adjacent deck surfaces.

6.5.5   Deck Drainage

Provide sufficient deck drainage and design deck and SCUPPER drain lines in all FOOD SERVICE and warewash areas to prevent liquids from pooling on the decks. Do not use DECK SINKS as substitutes for DECK DRAINS.

6.5.6   Cross-drain Connections

Provide cross-drain connections to prevent pooling and spillage from the SCUPPER when the vessel is listing.

6.5.7   Coaming

If a nonremovable coaming is provided around a DECK DRAINS, ensure that the juncture with the deck is COVED. Integral COVING is not required.

6.6   Ramps

6.6.1   Installation

Install ramps over thresholds and ensure that they are easily REMOVABLE or sealed in place. Slope ramps for easy trolley roll-in and roll-out. Ensure ramps are strong enough to maintain their shape. If ramps over SCUPPER covers are built as an integral part of the SCUPPER system, construct them of SMOOTH, durable, and EASILY CLEANABLE materials.

6.7   Gray and Black Water Drain Lines

6.7.1   Installation

Limit the installation of drain lines that carry BLACK WATER or other liquid wastes directly overhead or horizontally through spaces used for FOOD PREPARATION or STORAGE. This limitation includes areas for washing or storing utensils and equipment (e.g., in bars, in deck pantries, and over buffet counters).

If installation of waste lines is unavoidable in these areas, sleeve weld or butt weld steel piping; and heat fuse or chemically weld plastic piping.

For SCUPPER lines, factory assembled transition fittings for steel to plastic pipes are allowed when manufactured per ASTM F1973 or equivalent standard. Do not use push-fit or press-fit piping over these areas.

7.0 General Hygiene Facilities Requirements for Food Areas

7.1 Handwashing Stations

7.1.1 Potable Water

Provide hot and cold POTABLE WATER to all handwashing sinks.

Equip handwashing sinks to provide water at a temperature between 38°C (100°F) and 49°C (120°F) through a mixing valve or combination faucet.

7.1.2 Construction

Construct handwashing sinks of stainless steel in FOOD AREAS. Handwashing sinks in FOOD SERVICE AREAS and bars may be constructed of a similar, SMOOTH, durable material.

7.1.3 Supplies

Provide handwashing stations that include a soap dispenser, paper towel dispenser, corrosion-resistant waste receptacle, and, where necessary, splash panels to protect
- adjoining equipment,
- clean utensils,
- FOOD STORAGE, or
- FOOD PREPARATION surfaces.

If attached to the bulkhead, permanently seal soap dispensers, paper towel dispensers, and waste towel receptacles or make them REMOVABLE for cleaning. Air hand dryers are not permitted.

7.1.4 Dispenser Locations

Install soap dispensers and paper towel dispensers so that they are not over adjoining equipment, clean utensil storage, FOOD STORAGE, FOOD PREPARATION surfaces, bar counters, or water fountains.

For a multiple-station sink, ensure that there is a soap dispenser within 380 millimeters (15 inches) of each faucet and a paper towel dispenser within 760 millimeters (30 inches) of each faucet.

7.1.5 Dispenser Installation

Install paper towel dispensers a minimum of 450 millimeters (18 inches) above the deck (as measured from the lower edge of the dispenser).

7.1.6 Installation Specifications

Install handwash sinks a minimum of 750 millimeters (30 inches) above the deck, as measured at the top edge of the basin, and so that employees do not have to reach excessively to wash their hands.

Install counter-mounted handwash sinks a minimum of 600 millimeters

(24 inches) above the deck, as measured at the counter level.

The minimum size of the handwash sink basin must be 300 millimeters (12 inches) in length and 300 millimeters (12 inches) in width. The diameter of round basins must be at least 300 millimeters (12 inches). Additionally, the minimum distance from the bottom of the water tap to the bottom of the basin must be 200 millimeters (8 inches).

7.1.7 Locations

Locate handwashing stations throughout FOOD-HANDLING, PREPARATION, and warewash areas so that no employee must walk more than 8 meters (26 feet) to reach a station or pass through a normally closed door that requires touching a handle to open.

7.1.7.1 *Food-dispensing Waiter Stations*

Provide a handwashing station at food-dispensing waiter stations (e.g., soups, ice, etc.) where the staff do not routinely return to an area with a handwashing station.

7.1.7.2 *Food-handling Areas*

Provide a handwashing station in provision areas where bulk raw foods are handled by provisioning staff.

7.1.7.3 *Crew Buffets*

Provide at least one handwashing station for every 100 seats (e.g., 1–100 seats = one handwashing station, 101–200 seats = two handwashing stations, etc.). Locate stations near the entrance of all officer/staff/crew mess areas where FOOD SERVICE lines are "self-service."

7.1.7.4 *Soiled Dish Drop-off*

Install handwashing stations at the soiled dish drop-off area(s) in the main galley, specialty galleys, and pantries for employees bringing soiled dishware from the dining rooms or other FOOD SERVICE AREAS to prevent long waiting lines at handwashing stations. Provide one sink or one faucet on a multiple-station sink for every 10 wait staff who handle clean items and are assigned to a FOOD SERVICE AREA during maximum capacity.

During the plan review, VSP will evaluate work assignments for wait staff to determine the appropriate number of handwashing stations.

7.1.8 Faucet Handles

Install easy-to-operate sanitary faucet handles (e.g., large elephant-ear handles, foot pedals, knee pedals, or electronic sensors) on handwashing sinks in FOOD AREAS. If a faucet is self-closing, slow-closing, or metering, provide a water flow of at least 15 seconds without the need to reactivate the faucet.

7.1.9 Signs

Install permanent signs in English and other appropriate languages stating "wash hands often," "wash hands frequently," or similar wording.

7.2 Bucket Filling Station

7.2.1 Location

Provide at least one bucket filling station in each area of the galleys (e.g., cold galley, hot galley, bakery, etc.), FOOD STORAGE, and FOOD PREPARATION AREAS.

7.2.2 Mixing Valve

Supply hot and cold POTABLE WATER through a mixing valve to a faucet with the appropriate BACKFLOW protection at each bucket filling station.

7.2.3 Deck Drainage

Provide appropriate deck drainage (e.g., SCUPPER or sloping deck to DECK DRAIN) under all bucket filling stations to eliminate any pooling of water on the decks below the bucket filling station.

7.3 Crew Public Toilet Rooms for Food Service Employees

7.3.1 Location and Number

Install at least one employee toilet room in close proximity to the work area of all FOOD PREPARATION AREAS (beverage-only service bars are excluded). Provide one toilet per 25 employees and provide separate facilities for males and females if more than 25 employees are assigned to a FOOD PREPARATION AREA, excluding wait staff. This refers to the shift with the maximum number of food employees, excluding wait staff. Urinals may be installed, but do not count toward the toilet/employee ratio.

7.3.1.1 Main Galleys and Crew Galleys

For main galleys and crew galleys, locate toilet rooms inside the FOOD PREPARATION AREA or in a passageway immediately outside the area. If a main galley has multiple levels and there is stairwell access between the galleys, toilet rooms may be located near the stairwell within one deck above or below.

7.3.1.2 Other Food Service Outlets

For other FOOD SERVICE outlets (lido galley, specialty galley, etc.), do not locate toilet rooms more than two decks above/below within the distance of a fire zone, if on the same deck, no more than one fire zone away (should be within the same fire zone or an adjacent fire zone). If more than one FOOD SERVICE outlet is located on the same deck, the toilet room may be located on the same deck between the outlets and within two fire zones of each outlet.

7.3.1.3   *Provisions*

For preparations rooms located in provisions areas, use the distance requirement described in 7.3.1.2 to locate toilet rooms.

7.3.2   Ventilation and Handwashing

Install exhaust ventilation and handwashing facilities in each toilet room. Air hand dryers are not permitted in these toilet rooms. Install a permanent sign in English, and other languages where appropriate, stating the exact wording: "WASH HANDS AFTER USING THE TOILET." Locate this sign on the bulkhead adjacent to the main toilet room door or on the main door inside the toilet room.

7.3.3   Hands-free Exit

Ensure hands-free exit for toilet rooms, as described in section 36.1.1. Ensure handwashing facilities have sanitary faucet handles as in section 7.1.8.

7.3.4   Doors

Install tight-fitting, self-closing doors.

7.3.5   Decks

Construct decks of hard, durable materials and provide COVING at the bulkhead-deck juncture.

7.3.6   Deckheads and Bulkheads

Install EASILY CLEANABLE deckheads and bulkheads.

8.0   Equipment Placement and Mounting

8.1   Seal

Seal counter-mounted equipment that is not PORTABLE to the bulkhead, tabletop, countertop, or adjacent equipment.

If the equipment is not sealed, provide sufficient, unobstructed space for cleaning around, behind, and between fixed equipment. The space provided is dependent on the distance from either a position directly in front or from either side of the equipment to the farthest point requiring cleaning as described in sections 8.1.1 through 8.1.4 below. These requirements do not apply to open racks, other equipment of open design, or PORTABLE equipment. See also Figures 8a through 8d.

8.1.1   Cleaning Distance Less Than 600 Millimeters (24 Inches)

A distance to be cleaned of less than 600 millimeters (24 inches) requires an unobstructed space of 150 millimeters (6 inches).

8.1.2   Cleaning Distance Between 600 Millimeters (24 Inches) and 1,200 Millimeters (48 Inches)

A distance to be cleaned between 600 millimeters (24 inches) and

1,200 millimeters (48 inches) requires an unobstructed space of 200 millimeters (8 inches).

8.1.3 Cleaning Distance Between 1,200 Millimeters (48 Inches) and 1,800 Millimeters (72 Inches)

A distance to be cleaned between 1,200 millimeters (48 inches) and 1,800 millimeters (72 inches) requires an unobstructed space of 300 millimeters (12 inches).

8.1.4 Cleaning Distance Greater Than 1,800 Millimeters (72 Inches)

A distance to be cleaned greater than 1,800 millimeters (72 inches) requires an unobstructed space of 460 millimeters (18 inches).

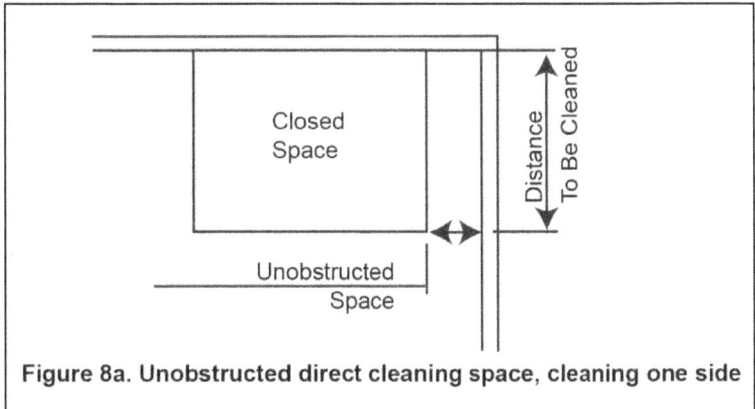

Figure 8a. Unobstructed direct cleaning space, cleaning one side

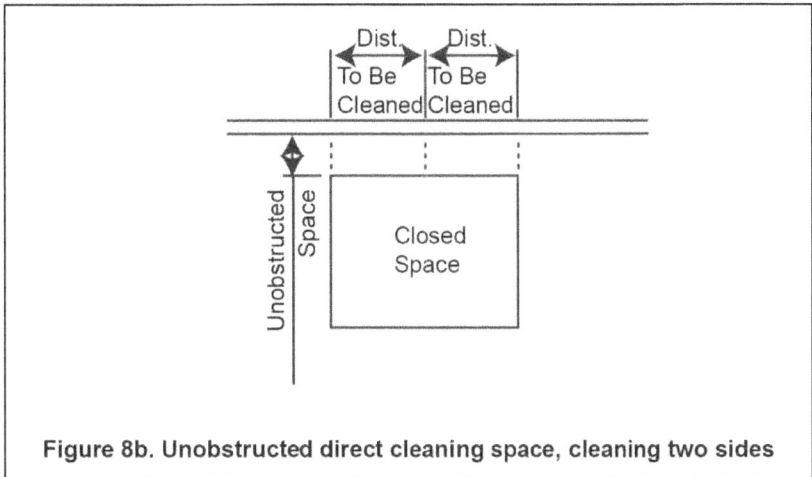

Figure 8b. Unobstructed direct cleaning space, cleaning two sides

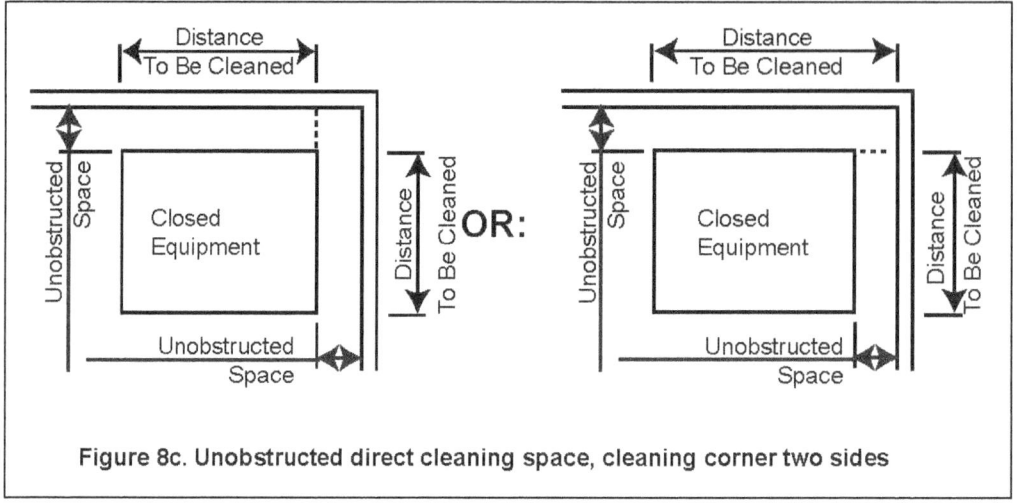

Figure 8c. Unobstructed direct cleaning space, cleaning corner two sides

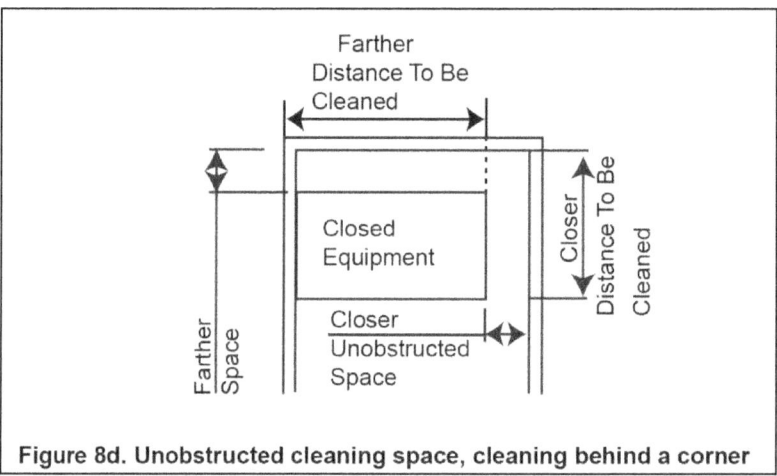

Figure 8d. Unobstructed cleaning space, cleaning behind a corner

8.1.5   Cleaning Distance

In case the unobstructed cleaning space includes a corner, the cleaning distance has to be treated separately in two sections. The farther space behind the equipment has to be treated separately according to sections 8.1.1 through 8.1.4. The closer space beside the equipment has to be treated by calculating closer and farther cleaning distance together and using cleaning space according to sections 8.1.1 through 8.1.4. The closer space always has to be minimum of 300 millimeters (12 inches). See Figure 8d.

8.2   Seal or Elevate

Seal equipment that is not PORTABLE to the deck or elevate it on legs that provide at least a 150-millimeter (6-inch) clearance between the deck and the equipment. If no part of the equipment is more than 150 millimeters (6 inches) from the point of cleaning access, the clearance space may be only 100 millimeters (4 inches). This includes vending and dispensing machines in FOOD AREAS, including mess rooms.

Exceptions to the equipment requirements may be granted if there are no barriers to cleaning (e.g., equipment such as waste handling systems and warewashing machines with pipelines, motors, and cables) where a 150-millimeter (6-inch) clearance from the deck may not be practical.

8.2.1 Deck Mounting

Continuous weld all equipment that is not PORTABLE to stainless steel pads or plates on the deck. Ensure the welds have SMOOTH edges, rounded corners, and no GAPS.

8.2.2 Adhesives

Attach deck-mounted equipment as an integral part of the deck surface with glue, epoxy, or other durable, APPROVED adhesive product. Ensure that the attached surfaces are SMOOTH and EASILY CLEANABLE.

8.3 Deckhead Clearance

Provide a minimum of at least 150 millimeters (6 inches) between equipment and deckheads. If this clearance cannot be achieved, extend the equipment to the deckhead panels and seal appropriately.

8.4 Foundation or Coaming

Provide a sealed-type foundation or coaming for equipment not mounted on legs. Do not allow equipment to overhang the foundation or coaming by more than 100 millimeters (4 inches). Completely seal any overhanging equipment along the bottom (Figure 9).

Mount equipment that is on a foundation or coaming at least 100 millimeters (4 inches) above the finished deck. Use cement, hard SEALANT, or continuous weld to seal equipment to the foundation or coaming.

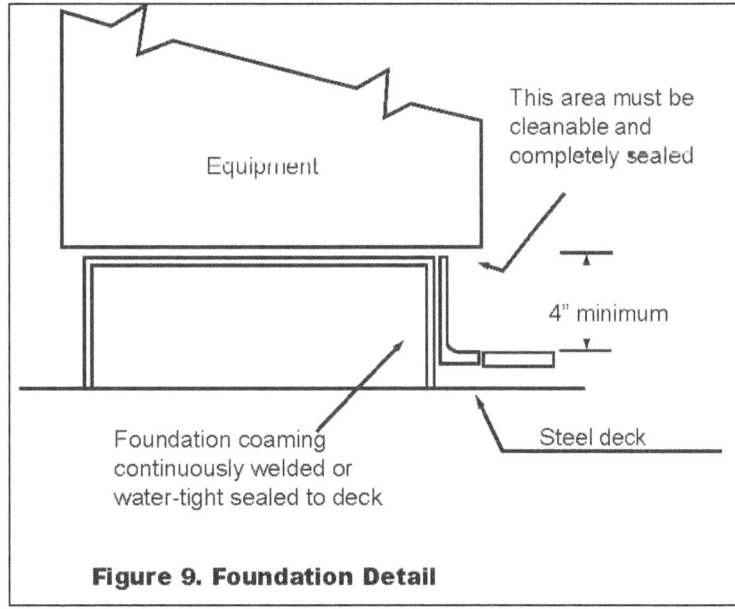

Figure 9. Foundation Detail

8.5   Counter-Mounted Equipment

Seal counter-mounted equipment, unless PORTABLE, to the countertop or mount on legs.

8.5.1   Leg Length

The length of the legs is dependent on the horizontal distance of the table top under the equipment from either end to the farthest point requiring cleaning, based on the table below.

Horizontal Distance (depth)	Equipment Leg Length
> 750 millimeters (30 inches)	At least 150 millimeters (6 inches)
500 to 750 millimeters (20 to 30 inches)	At least 100 millimeters (4 inches)
75 to 500 millimeters (3 to 20 inches)	At least 75 millimeters (3 inches)
Less than 75 millimeters (3 inches)	50 millimeters (2 inches)

9.0   Fasteners and Requirements for Securing and Sealing Equipment

9.1   Food-contact Surfaces

9.1.1   Attach

Attach all FOOD-CONTACT SURFACES or connections from FOOD-CONTACT SURFACES to adjacent splash zones to ensure a seamless COVED corner.

Reinforce all bulkheads, deckheads, or decks receiving such attachments.

9.1.2   Fasteners

Use low profile, nonslotted, NONCORRODING, and easy-to-clean fasteners on FOOD-CONTACT SURFACES and in splash zones. The use of exposed slotted screws, Phillips head screws, or pop rivets in these areas is prohibited.

9.2   Nonfood-contact Surfaces

9.2.1   Seal

Seal equipment SEAMS with an appropriate SEALANT (see SEAM definition). Avoid excessive use of SEALANT.

Use stainless steel profile strips on surfaces exposed to extreme temperatures (e.g., freezers, cook tops, grills, and fryers) or for GAPS greater than 3 millimeters (1/8 inch). Do not use SEALANTS to close GAPS.

9.2.2 Fasteners

Construct slotted or Phillips head screws, pop rivets, and other fasteners used in NONFOOD-CONTACT AREAS of NONCORRODING materials.

9.3 Use of Sealants

9.3.1 Approved

Use APPROVED (certified to ANSI/NSF Standard 51 or equivalent criteria) food grade SEALANTS on FOOD-CONTACT SURFACES. Avoid excessive use of SEALANT. Once cured, SEALANTS must be SMOOTH, semihard or hard, durable and easy to clean. Soft SEALANTS can be used in ice machines. Provide product manufacturers' literature and certification listing for SEALANTS used.

10.0 Latches, Hinges, and Handles

10.1 Durable, Noncorroding, and Easily Cleanable

Use durable, NONCORRODING, and EASILY CLEANABLE built-in equipment latches, hinges, and handles. Do not use piano hinges in FOOD-CONTACT SURFACES.

11.0 Gaskets

11.1 Materials

Use SMOOTH, nonabsorbent, nonporous materials for equipment gaskets in reach-in refrigerators, steamers, ice bins, ice cream freezers, and similar equipment.

11.2 Exposed Surfaces

Close and seal exposed surfaces of gaskets at their ends and corners.

11.3 Removable

Use refrigerator door gaskets that are designed to be REMOVABLE.

11.4 Fasteners

Follow the requirements in section 9.0 when using fasteners to install gaskets.

12.0 Equipment Drain Lines

12.1 Connections

Connect drain lines to the appropriate waste system by means of an AIR GAP or AIR-BREAK from all fixtures, sinks, appliances, compartments, refrigeration units, or other equipment used, designed for, or intended to be used in the preparation, processing, storage, or handling of food, ice, or drinks. Ensure that the AIR GAP or AIR-BREAK is easily ACCESSIBLE for inspection and cleaning.

12.2   Construction Materials

Use stainless steel or other durable, NONCORRODING, and EASILY CLEANABLE rigid or flexible material in the construction of drain lines. Do not use ribbed, braided, or woven materials in areas subject to splash or soiling unless coated with a SMOOTH, durable, and EASILY CLEANABLE material.

12.3   Size

Size drain lines appropriately, with a minimum interior diameter of 25 millimeters (1 inch) for custom-built equipment.

12.4   Walk-in Refrigerators and Freezers

Slope walk-in refrigerator and freezer evaporator drain lines and extend them through the bulkhead or deck.

12.4.1   Evaporator Drain Lines

Direct walk-in refrigerator and freezer evaporator drain lines through an ACCESSIBLE AIR-BREAK to a deck SCUPPER or drain below the deck level or to a SCUPPER outside the unit.

12.4.2   Deck Drains and Scuppers

Direct drain lines from DECK DRAINS and SCUPPERS in walk-in refrigerator and freezer units through an indirect connection to the wastewater system.

12.5   Horizontal Distance

Install drain lines to minimize the horizontal distance from the source of the drainage to the discharge.

12.6   Vertical Distance

Install horizontal drain lines at least 100 millimeters (4 inches) above the deck and slope to drain.

12.7   Food Equipment Drain Lines

All drain lines (except condensate drain lines) from hood washing systems, cold-top tables, bains-marie, dipper wells, UTILITY SINKS, and warewashing sinks or machines must meet the following criteria:

12.7.1   Length

Lines must be less than 1,000 millimeters (40 inches) in length and free of sharp angles or corners if designed to be cleaned in place by a brush.

12.7.2   Cleaning

Lines must be READILY REMOVABLE for cleaning if they are longer than 1,000 millimeters (40 inches).

12.7.3   Extend Vertically

Extend fixed equipment drain lines vertically to a SCUPPER or DECK DRAIN when possible. If not possible, keep the horizontal distance of the line to a minimum.

12.7.4 Air-break

Handwashing sinks, mop sinks, and drinking fountains are not required to drain through an AIR-BREAK.

13.0 Electrical Connections, Pipelines, Service Lines, and Attached Equipment

13.1 Encase

Encase electrical wiring from permanently installed equipment in durable and EASILY CLEANABLE material. Do not use ribbed or woven stainless steel electrical conduit where it is subject to splash or soiling unless it is encased in EASILY CLEANABLE plastic or similar EASILY CLEANABLE material. Do not use ribbed, braided, or woven conduit.

13.2 Install or Fasten

For equipment that is not permanently mounted, install or fasten service lines in a manner that prevents the lines from contacting decks or countertops.

13.3 Mounted Equipment

Tightly seal bulkhead or deckhead-mounted equipment (phones, speakers, electrical control panels, outlet boxes, etc.) with the bulkhead or deckhead panels. Do not locate such equipment in areas exposed to food splash.

13.4 Seal Penetrations

Tightly seal any areas where electrical lines, steam or water pipelines, etc., penetrate the panels or tiles of the deck, bulkhead, or deckhead, including inside technical spaces located above or below equipment or work surfaces. Seal any openings or voids around the electrical lines or the steam or water pipelines and the surrounding conduit or pipelines.

13.5 Enclose Pipelines

Enclose steam and water pipelines to kettles and boilers in stainless steel cabinets or position the pipelines behind bulkhead panels. Minimize the number of exposed pipelines. Cover any exposed insulated pipelines with stainless steel or other durable, EASILY CLEANABLE material.

14.0 Hood Systems

14.1 Warewashing

Install canopy exhaust hood or direct duct exhaust systems over warewashing equipment (except undercounter warewashing machines) and over three-compartment sinks in pot wash areas where hot water is used for sanitizing.

14.1.1 Direct Duct Exhaust

Directly connect warewashing machines that have a direct duct exhaust to the hood exhaust trunk.

14.1.2 Overhang

Provide canopy exhaust hoods over warewashing equipment or three-compartment sinks to have a minimum 150-millimeter (6-inch) overhang from the edge of equipment to capture excess steam and heat and prevent condensate from collecting on surfaces.

14.1.3 Cleanout Ports

Install cleanout ports in the direct exhaust ducts of the ventilation systems between the top of the warewashing machine and the hood system or deckhead.

14.1.4 Drip Trays

Provide ACCESSIBLE and REMOVABLE condensate DRIP TRAYS in warewashing machine ventilation ducts.

14.2 Cooking and Hot Holding Equipment

14.2.1 Cooking Equipment

Install hood or canopy systems above cooking equipment in accordance with safety of life-at-sea (SOLAS) requirements to ensure that they remove excess steam and grease-laden vapors and prevent condensate from collecting on surfaces.

14.2.2 Hot Holding Equipment

Install a hood or canopy system or dedicated local exhaust ventilation directly above bains marie, steam tables, or other open hot holding equipment to control excess heat and steam and prevent condensate from collecting on surfaces.

14.2.3 Countertop and Portable Equipment

Install a hood or canopy system or dedicated local extraction when SOLAS requirements do not specify an exhaust system for countertop cooking appliances or where PORTABLE appliances are used. The exhaust system must remove excess steam and grease-laden vapors and prevent collection of the cooking byproducts or condensate on surfaces.

14.3 Size

Properly size all exhaust and supply vents.

14.3.1 Position and Balance

Position and balance all exhaust and supply vents to ensure proper air conditioning and capture/exhaust of heat and steam.

14.3.2 Prevent Condensate

Limit condensate formation on either the exhaust canopy hood or air supply vents by either:
- locating or directing conditioned air away from exhaust hoods and heat generating equipment or
- installing a shield blocking the air from the hood supply vents.

14.4 Filters

Where used, provide READILY REMOVABLE and cleanable filters.

14.5 Access

Provide access for cleaning vents and ductwork. Automatic clean-in-place systems are recommended for removal of grease generated from cooking equipment.

14.6 Hood Cleaning Cabinets

Locate automatic clean-in-place hood wash control panels that have a chemical reservoir so they are not over FOOD PREPARATION equipment or counters, FOOD PREPARATION or warewashing sinks, or food and clean equipment storage.

14.7 Construction

Construct hood systems of stainless steel with COVED corners of at least a 9.5-millimeter (3/8-inch) radius.

14.7.1 Continuous Welds

Use continuous welds or profile strips on adjoining pieces of stainless steel.

14.7.2 Drainage System

Install a drainage system for automatic clean-in-place hood-washing systems.

A drainage system is not required for normal grease and condensate hoods or for locations where cleaning solutions are applied manually to hood assemblies.

14.8 Manufacturer's Recommendations

Install all ventilation systems in accordance with the manufacturer's recommendations.

14.8.1 Test System

Test each system using a method that determines if the system is properly balanced for normal operating conditions. Provide written documentation of the test results.

15.0 Provision Rooms, Walk-in Refrigerators and Freezers, and Food Transportation Corridors

15.1   Bulkheads and Deckheads

15.1.1   Refrigerators and Freezers
Provide tight-fitting stainless steel bulkheads in walk-in refrigerators and freezers. Line doors with stainless steel.

15.1.2   Food Transportation Corridors
Light-colored painted steel is acceptable for provision passageways and FOOD TRANSPORTATION CORRIDORS. However, FOOD TRANSPORTATION CORRIDORS inside galleys must be built to galley standards (see section 16.0).

15.1.3   Difficult-to-clean Equipment
- Close deckhead-mounted cable trays, piping, or other difficult-to-clean deckhead-mounted equipment or
- Close the deckhead to prevent food contamination from dust and debris falling from deckheads and deckhead-mounted equipment and utilities.

Painted sheet metal ceilings are acceptable in these areas.

15.1.4   Dry Storage
Stainless steel panels are preferable but not required in DRY STORAGE AREAS.

15.1.5   Protection
Provide protection to prevent damage to bulkheads from pallet handling equipment (e.g., forklifts, pallet jacks, etc.) in areas through which food is stored or transferred.

15.2   Decks

15.2.1   Materials
Use hard, durable, nonabsorbent decking (e.g., tiles or diamond-plate corrugated stainless steel deck panels) in refrigerated provision rooms. Install durable COVING as an integral part of the deck and bulkhead interface and at the juncture between decks and equipment foundations. Sufficiently reinforce stainless steel decking to prevent buckling if pallet handling equipment will be used in these areas.

15.2.2   Steel Decking
Steel decking is acceptable in provision passageways, FOOD TRANSPORTATION

CORRIDORS, and DRY STORAGE AREAS. However, FOOD TRANSPORTATION CORRIDORS inside galleys must be built to galley standards (see section 16.0).

15.3 Cold Room Evaporators, Drip Pan, and Drain Lines

15.3.1 Enclose Components

Enclose piping, wiring, coils, and other difficult-to-clean components of evaporators in walk-in refrigerators, freezers, and DRY STORAGE AREAS with stainless steel panels.

15.3.2 Fasteners

Follow all fastener guidelines in section 9.0.

15.3.3 Drip Pans

15.3.3.1 Materials

Use stainless steel evaporator drip pans that have COVED corners, are sloped to drain, are strong enough to maintain slope, and are ACCESSIBLE for cleaning.

15.3.3.2 Spacers

Place NONCORRODING spacers between the drip pan brackets and the interior edges of the pans.

15.3.3.3 Heater Coil

Provide a heater coil for freezer drip pans. Attach the coil to a stainless steel insert panel or to the underside of the drip pan. Use easily REMOVABLE coils so that the drip pan can be cleaned. Make sure that heating coils provided for drain lines are installed inside of the lines.

15.3.3.4 Position and Size

Position and size the evaporator drip pan to collect all condensate dripping from the evaporator unit.

15.3.4 Thermometer Probes

Encase thermometer probes in a stainless steel conduit. Position probes in the warmest part of the room where food is normally stored. These probes are for monitoring the internal air temperature only.

16.0 Galleys, Food Preparation Rooms, and Pantries

16.1 Bulkheads and Deckheads

16.1.1 Construction

Construct bulkheads and deckheads (including doors, door frames, and columns) with a high-quality corrosion-resistant stainless steel. Use a thick enough gauge so that the panels do not warp, flex, or separate under normal conditions. Use an appropriate SEALANT for SEAMS. Use stainless steel or other NONCORRODING, but equally durable, materials for profile strips on bulkhead and deckhead GAPS.

16.1.1.1 *Gaps*
Minimize GAPS around fire shutters, sliding doors, and pass-through windows.

16.1.1.2 *Access Panels*
Provide sufficiently sized access panels to void spaces around sliding doors and sliding pass-through windows to allow for cleaning.

16.1.2 Sufficient Thickness
Construct bulkheads of sufficient thickness or reinforce the areas where equipment is installed to allow the use of fasteners or welding without compromising the quality and construction of the panels.

16.1.3 Utility Lines
Install utility line connections through a stainless steel or other EASILY CLEANABLE conduit that is mounted away from bulkheads and deckheads.

16.1.4 Backsplashes
Attach backsplashes to the bulkhead with low profile nonslotted fasteners or with continuous welds and tack welds that are polished SMOOTH. Use an appropriate SEALANT to make the backsplash attachment watertight.

16.1.5 Penetrations
Close all openings where piping and other items penetrate the bulkheads and deckheads, including inside technical compartments.

16.2 Decks

16.2.1 Construction
Construct decks from hard, durable, nonabsorbent, nonskid material. Install durable COVING
- As an integral part of the deck and bulkhead interface,
- At the juncture between decks and equipment foundations, and
- Between the deck and equipment.

16.2.2 Seal Tiling
Seal all deck tiling with a durable watertight grouting material. Seal stainless steel deck plate panels with a continuous NONCORRODING weld.

16.2.3 Technical Compartments
Use durable, nonabsorbent, EASILY CLEANABLE surfaces such as tile or stainless steel in technical spaces below undercounter cabinets, counters, or refrigerators. Do not use painted steel and concrete decking.

16.2.4 Penetrations

Seal all openings where piping and other items penetrate through the deck.

17.0 Buffet Lines, Waiter Stations, Bars, and Other Similar Food Service Areas

Follow construction guidelines referenced in sections 6.0 through 16.2.4 for all pantries.

17.1 Bulkheads and Deckheads

17.1.1 Construction

Construct bulkheads and deckheads of hard, durable, NONCORRODING, nonabsorbent and EASILY CLEANABLE materials.

Deckheads must be provided above all buffet lines, waiter stations, bars, and other similar FOOD SERVICE AREAS.

17.1.2 Ventilation Slots

Slots for ventilation plenum spaces are not allowed directly over FOOD PREPARATION, FOOD STORAGE, or clean equipment storage.

17.1.3 Buffet Service Areas

For buffet service areas where FOOD PREPARATION occurs, galley standards for construction must be followed (see section 16.0). FOOD PREPARATION AREAS include areas where utensils are used to mix and prepare foods (e.g., salad, sandwich, sushi, pizza, meat carving) and the food is prepared and cooked (e.g., grills, ovens, fryers, griddles, skillets, waffle makers).

If such facilities are installed along a buffet counter, they will be evaluated in the plan review. For example, a station specific for salads, sushi, deli, or a pizzeria is a preparation area, as are locations where foods are prepared completely (e.g., waffle batter poured into griddle, cooked, plated, and served). However, a one-person carving station is not a preparation area. Omelet stations would have to be evaluated.

17.2 Decks

17.2.1 Buffet Lines

Install hard, durable, nonabsorbent, nonskid decks at all buffet lines that are at least 1,000 millimeters (40 inches) in width measured from the edge of the service counter or, if present, from the outside edge of the tray rail. Carpet, vinyl, and linoleum deck materials are not acceptable.

17.2.2 Waiter Stations

Install hard, durable, nonabsorbent decks (e.g., tile, sealed granite, or marble) that extend at least 600 millimeters (24 inches) from the edge of the working side(s) of the waiter stations. The sides of stations that have a splash shield of 150 millimeters (6 inches) or higher are not considered working sides. Carpet, vinyl, and linoleum deck materials are not acceptable.

17.2.3   Technical Spaces

Construct decks in technical spaces of hard, durable, nonabsorbent materials (e.g., tiles, epoxy resin, or stainless steel) and provide COVING. Do not use painted steel or concrete decking.

17.2.4   Worker Side of Buffets and Bars

Install durable COVING as an integral part of the deck/bulkhead and deck/cabinet foundation juncture on the worker-only side of the deck/buffet and deck/bar.

17.2.5   Consumer Side of Buffets and Waiter Stations

Install durable COVING at the consumer side of buffet service counters, counters shared with worker activities (islands), and waiter stations. Install durable COVING at deck/bulkhead junctures located within one meter of the waiter stations. Consumer sides of bars are excluded. See Figures 10a and 10b.

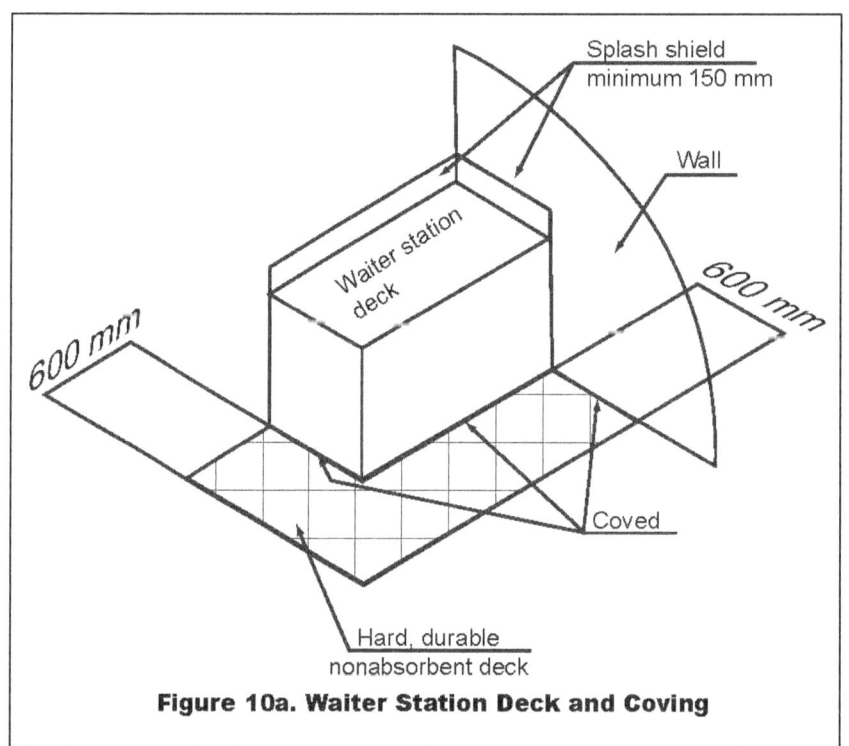

Figure 10a. Waiter Station Deck and Coving

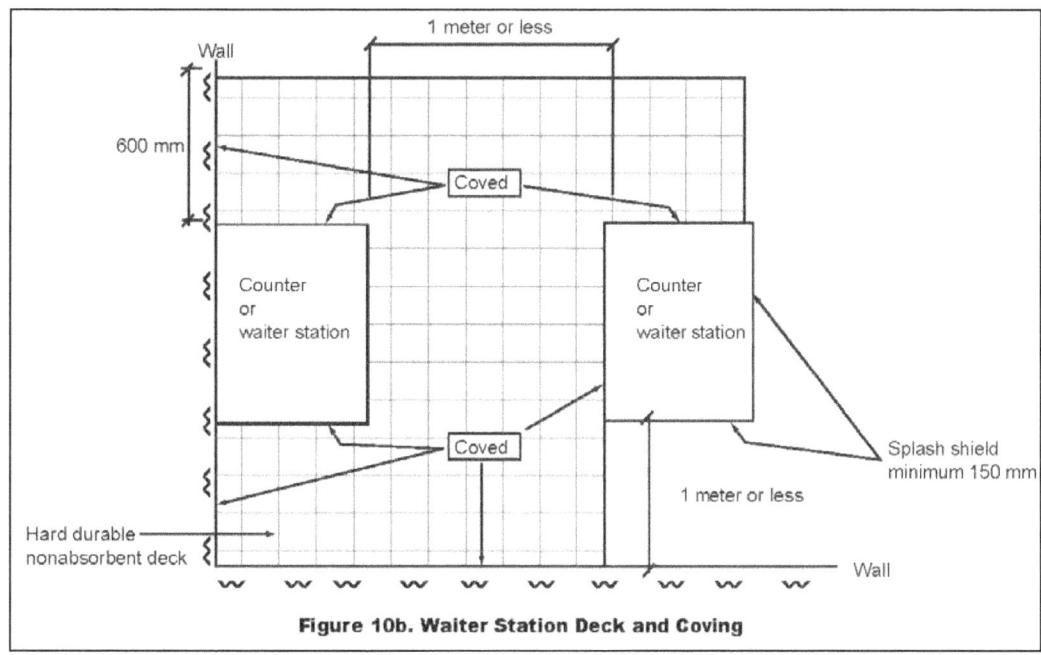

Figure 10b. Waiter Station Deck and Coving

17.2.6   Areas for Buffet Service and Food Preparation

For buffet service areas where FOOD PREPARATION occurs, galley standards for construction must be followed (see section 16.0).

17.3   Food Display Protection

17.3.1   Effective Means

Provide effective means to protect food (e.g., sneeze guards, display cases, raised shield) in all areas where food is on display. This includes locations where food is being displayed during preparation (e.g., carving stations, induction cooking stations, sushi, deli). This excludes teppanyaki style cooking.

17.3.1.1   Solid Vertical Shield Without Tray Rail

For a solid vertical shield without a tray rail, the minimum height from the deck to the top edge of the shield must be 140 centimeters.

17.3.1.2   Solid Vertical Shield With Tray Rail

For a solid vertical shield with a tray rail, for every 3 centimeters that the tray rail extends from the buffet, the height of the shield may be lowered by 1 centimeter, but the minimum height from the deck to the top edge of the shield must be 120 centimeters.

17.3.1.3   Consumer Seating at Counter

For designs where consumers are seated at the counter and workers are preparing food on the other side of the sneeze guard, consideration must be given to the height of the preparation counter, consumer counter, and consumer seat.

VSP will evaluate these designs and establish the shield height during the plan review.

17.3.2 Sneeze Guard Criteria

17.3.2.1 Portable or Built-in
Sneeze guards may be temporary (PORTABLE) or built-in and integral parts of display tables, bains marie, or cold-top tables.

17.3.2.2 Panel Material
Sneeze guard panels must be durable plastic or glass that is SMOOTH and EASILY CLEANABLE. Design panels to be cleaned in place or, if REMOVABLE for cleaning, use sections that are manageable in weight and length.

Sneeze guard panels must be transparent and designed to minimize obstruction of the customer's view of the food. To protect against chipping, provide edge guards for glass panels. Sneeze guards for preparation-only protection do not need to be transparent.

17.3.2.3 Spaces or Openings
If there are spaces or openings greater than 25 millimeters (1 inch) along the length of the sneeze guard (such as between two pieces of the sneeze guard), ensure that there are no food wells, bains marie, etc., under the spaces or openings.

17.3.2.4 Position
Position sneeze guards so that the panels intercept a line between the average consumer's mouth and the displayed foods. Take into account factors such as the height of the FOOD DISPLAY counter, the presence or absence of a tray rail, and the distance between the edge of the display counter and the actual placement of the food (Figure 10).

17.3.2.5 Sneeze Guard Design
If the buffet is built to the calculations in Figure 11:

The maximum vertical distance between a counter top and the bottom leading edge of a sneeze guard must be 356 millimeters (14 inches).

The bottom leading edge of the sneeze guard must extend a minimum horizontal distance of 178 mm (7 inches) beyond the front inside edge of a food well.

The sum of a sneeze guard's protected horizontal plane (X) and its protected vertical plane (Y) must equal a minimum of 457 millimeters (18 inches) (Figure 10). Either X or Y may equal 0.

Install side protection for sneeze guards if the distance between exposed food and where people are expected to stand is less than 1 meter (40 inches).

See Figures 12-15 for additional examples of sneeze guards.

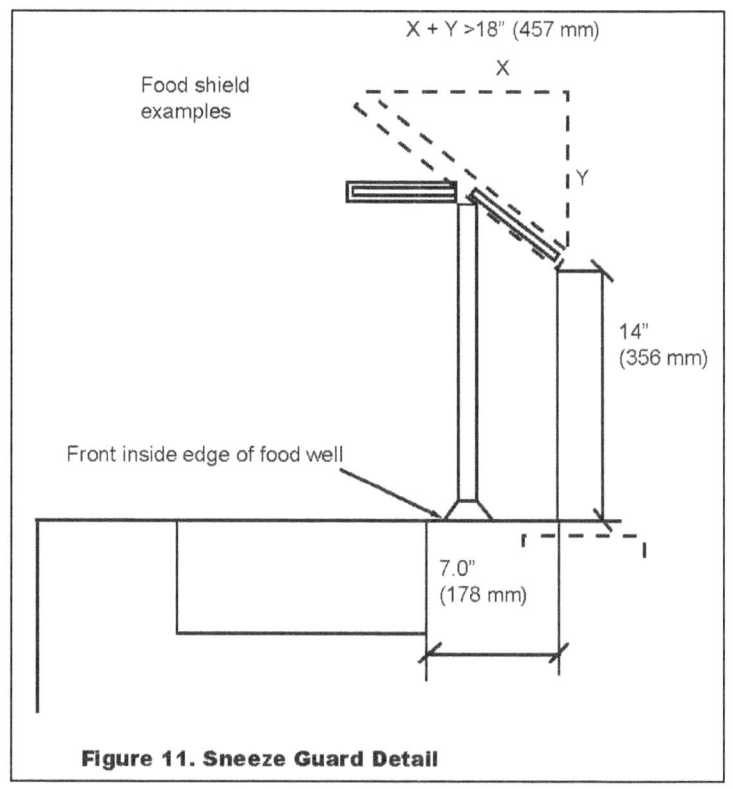

Figure 11. Sneeze Guard Detail

Food shield examples

X + Y >18" (457 mm)

X

Y

14" (356 mm)

Front inside edge of food well

7.0" (178 mm)

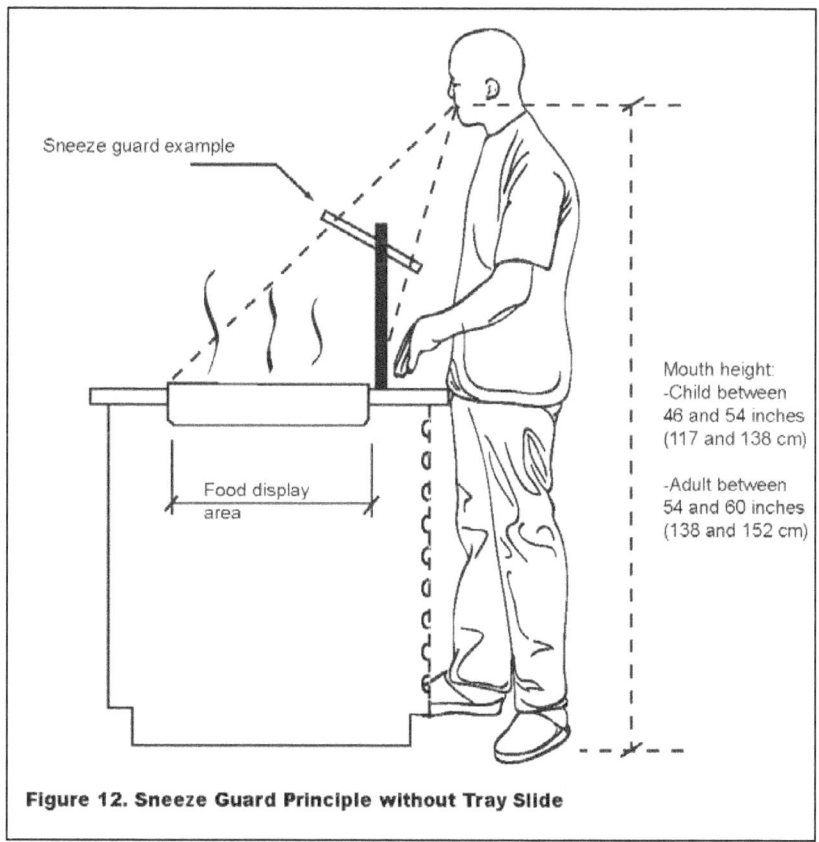

Sneeze guard example

Food display area

Mouth height:
-Child between 46 and 54 inches (117 and 138 cm)

-Adult between 54 and 60 inches (138 and 152 cm)

Figure 12. Sneeze Guard Principle without Tray Slide

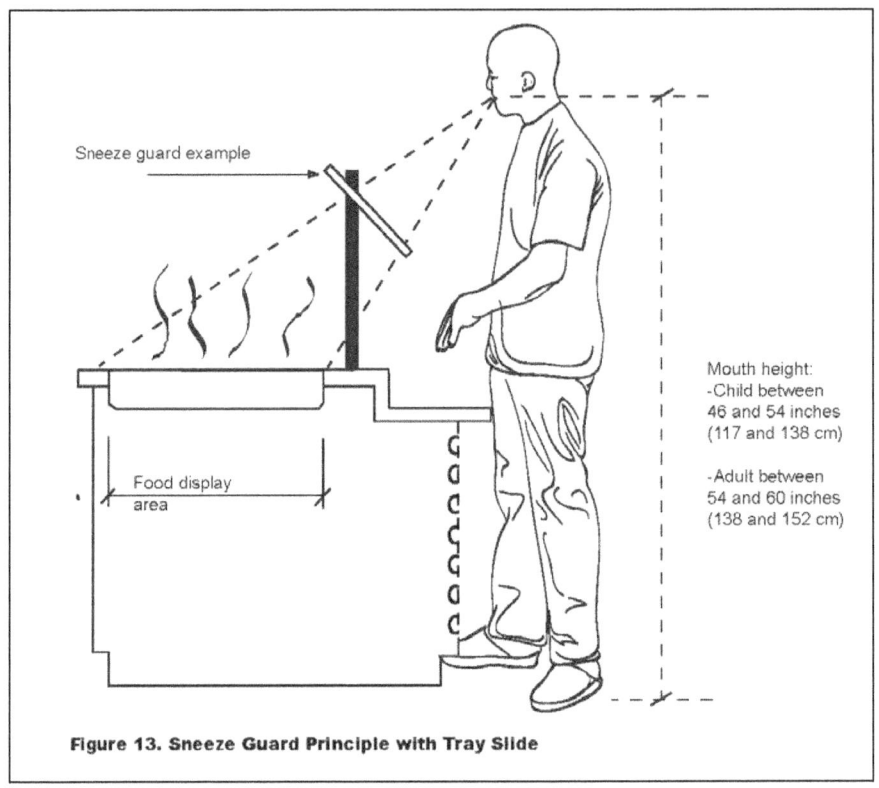

Sneeze guard example

Food display area

Mouth height:
-Child between
46 and 54 inches
(117 and 138 cm)

-Adult between
54 and 60 inches
(138 and 152 cm)

Figure 13. Sneeze Guard Principle with Tray Slide

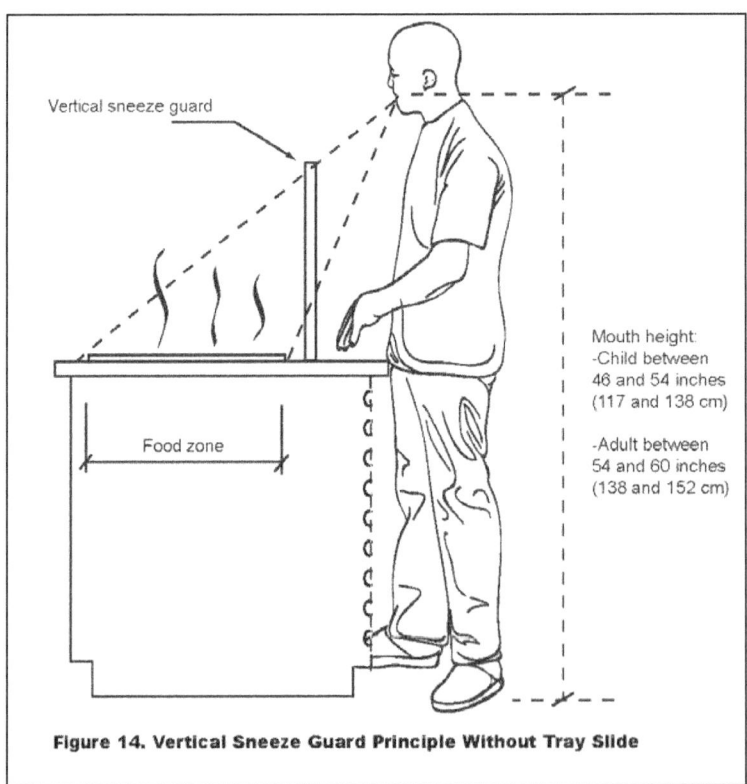

Vertical sneeze guard

Food zone

Mouth height:
-Child between
46 and 54 inches
(117 and 138 cm)

-Adult between
54 and 60 inches
(138 and 152 cm)

Figure 14. Vertical Sneeze Guard Principle Without Tray Slide

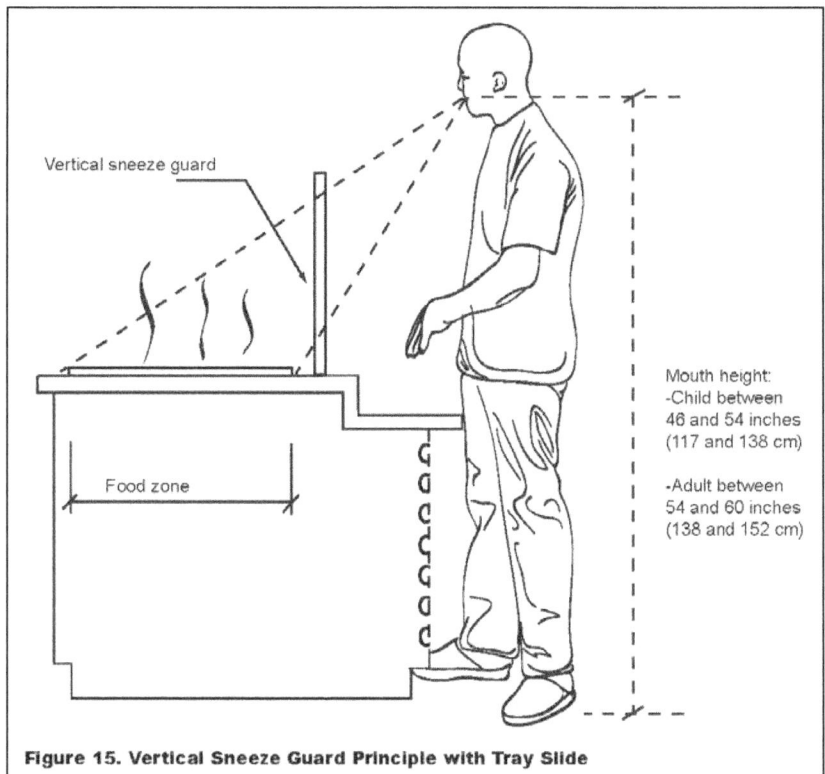

Figure 15. Vertical Sneeze Guard Principle with Tray Slide

Labels in figure: Vertical sneeze guard; Food zone; Mouth height: -Child between 46 and 54 inches (117 and 138 cm) -Adult between 54 and 60 inches (138 and 152 cm)

17.3.3   Tray Rail Surfaces

Use tray rail surfaces that are sealed, COVED, or have an open design. These surfaces must also be EASILY CLEANABLE in accordance with guidelines for food splash zones.

17.3.4   Food Pan Length

Consideration should be given to the length of the food pans in relation to the distance a consumer must reach to obtain food.

17.3.5   Soup Wells

If soups, oatmeal, and similar foods are to be self-served, equipment must be able to be placed under a sneeze guard.

17.4   Beverage Delivery System

17.4.1   Backflow Prevention Device

Install a BACKFLOW PREVENTION DEVICE that is APPROVED for use on carbonation systems (e.g., multiflow beverage dispensing systems). Install the device before the carbonator and downstream of brass or copper fittings in the POTABLE WATER supply line. A second device may be required if noncarbonated water is supplied to a multiflow hose dispensing gun.

17.4.2 Encase Supply Lines

Encase supply lines to the dispensing guns in a single tube. If the tube penetrates through any bulkhead or countertop, seal the penetration with a grommet.

17.4.3 Clean-in-place System

For bulk beverage delivery systems, incorporate fittings and connections for a clean-in-place system that can flush and sanitize the entire interior of the dispensing lines in accordance with the manufacturers' instructions.

17.5 Passenger Self-Service Buffet Handwashing Stations

17.5.1 Number

Provide one handwashing station per 100-passenger seating or fraction thereof. Stations should be equally distributed between the major passenger entry points to the buffet area and must be separate from a toilet room.

17.5.2 Passenger Entries

Provide handwashing stations at each minor passenger entry to the main buffet areas proportional to the passenger flow, with at least one per entry. These handwash stations can be counted towards the requirement of one per 100 passengers.

17.5.3 Self-service Stations Outside the Main Buffet

Provide at least one handwashing station at the passenger entrance of each self-service station outside of the main buffet. Beverage stations are excluded.

17.5.4 Equipment and Supplies

The handwashing station must include a handwash sink, soap dispenser, and single-use paper towel dispenser. Electric hand dryers can be installed in addition to paper towel dispensers. Waste receptacles must be provided in close proximity to the handwash sink and sized to accommodate the quantity of paper towel waste generated. The handwashing station may be decorative but must be nonabsorbent, durable, and EASILY CLEANABLE.

17.5.5 Automatic Handwashing System

An automatic handwashing system in lieu of a handwash sink is acceptable.

17.5.6 Sign

Each handwashing station must have a sign advising passengers to wash hands before eating. A pictogram can be used in lieu of words on the sign.

17.5.7 Location

Stations can be installed just outside of the entry. Position the handwashing stations along the passenger flow to the buffets.

17.5.8 Lighting

Provide a minimum of 110 lux lighting at the handwash stations.

17.6 Bar Counter Tops

17.6.1 Access

Bar counter tops are to be constructed to provide access for workers and to prevent workers from stooping or crawling to access the bar area from pantries or service areas.

18.0 Warewashing

18.1 Prewash Hoses

Provide rinse hoses for prewashing (not required but recommended in bar and deck pantries). If a sink is to be used for prerinsing, provide a REMOVABLE strainer.

18.1.1 Splash Panel

Install a splash panel if a clean utensil/glass storage rack or preparation counter is within an unobstructed 2 meters (6½ feet) of a prewash spray hose. This does not include the area behind the worker.

18.2 Food Waste Disposal

Provide space for trash cans, garbage grinder, or FOOD WASTE SYSTEMS. Grinders are optional in pantries and bars.

18.3 Trough

Provide a food waste trough that extends the full length of soiled landing tables with FOOD WASTE SYSTEMS.

18.4 Seal

Seal the back edge of the soiled landing table to the bulkhead or provide a minimum clearance between the table and the bulkhead according to section 8.0.

18.5 Design

Design soiled landing tables to drain waste liquids and prevent contamination of adjacent clean surfaces.

18.6 Drain and Slope

Provide across-the-counter gutters with drains and slope the clean landing tables to the gutters at the exit from the warewashing machines. If the first gutter does not effectively remove pooled water, install additional gutter(s) and drain line(s). Minimize the length of drain lines and, when possible, direct them in a straight line to the deck SCUPPER.

18.7 Space for Cleaning

Provide sufficient space for cleaning around and behind equipment (e.g., FOOD WASTE SYSTEMS and warewashing machines). Refer to section 8.0 for spacing requirements.

18.8 Enclose Wiring

Enclose FOOD WASTE SYSTEM wiring in a durable and easy to clean stainless steel or nonmetallic watertight conduit. Install all warewashing machine components at least 150 millimeters (6 inches) above the deck, except as noted in section 8.4.

18.9 Splash Panels

Construct REMOVABLE splash panels of stainless steel to protect the FOOD WASTE SYSTEM and technical areas.

18.10 Materials

Construct grinder cones, FOOD WASTE SYSTEM tables, and dish-landing tables from stainless steel with continuous welding. Construct platforms for supporting warewashing equipment from stainless steel.

18.11 Size

Size warewashing machines for their intended use and install them according to the manufacturer's recommendations.

18.12 Alarm

Equip warewashing machines with an audible or visual alarm that indicates if the sanitizing temperature or chemical sanitizer drop below the levels stated on the machine data plate.

18.13 Data Plate

Affix data plate so that the information is easy to read by the operator. The data plate must include the following information as provided by the manufacturer of the warewash machine:

18.13.1 Water Temperatures

Temperatures required for washing, rinsing (if applicable), and sanitizing.

18.13.2 Water Pressure

Pressure required for the fresh water sanitizing rinse unless the machine is designed to use only a pumped sanitizing rinse.

18.13.3 Conveyer Speed or Cycle Time

Conveyor speed in meters or feet per minute or minimum transit time for belt conveyor machines; minimum transit time for rack conveyor machines; or cycle time for stationary rack machines.

18.13.4 Chemical Concentration

Chemical concentration (if chemical sanitizers are used).

18.14 Manuals and Schematics

Warewash machine operating manuals and schematics of the internal BACKFLOW PREVENTION DEVICES must be provided.

18.15 Pot and Utensil Washing

Provide pot and utensil washing facilities as listed in section 6.2.2.

18.16 Three-compartment Sinks

Correctly size three-compartment warewashing and potwashing sinks for their intended use. Use sinks that are large enough to submerge the largest piece of equipment used in the area that is served. Use sinks that have COVED, continuously welded, integral internal corners.

18.16.1 Prevent Excessive Contamination

Install one of the following arrangements to prevent excessive contamination of rinse water with wash water splash:
- Gutter and drain: An across-the-counter gutter with a drain that divides the compartments. The gutter should extend the entire distance from the front edge of the counter to the backsplash.
- Splash shield: A splash shield at least 25 millimeters (1 inch) above the flood level rim of the sink between the compartments. The splash shield should extend the entire distance from the front edge of the counter to the backsplash;
- Overflow drain: An overflow drain in the wash compartment 100 millimeters (4 inches) below the flood level.

18.16.2 Hot Water Sanitizing Sinks

Equip hot water sanitizing sinks with an easy-to-read TEMPERATURE-MEASURING DEVICE, a utensil/equipment retrieval system (e.g., long-handled stainless steel hook or other retrieval system), a jacketed or coiled steam supply with a temperature control valve, or electric heating system.

18.17 Shelving

Provide sufficient shelving for storage of soiled and clean ware. Use open round tubular shelving or racks. Design overhead shelves to drain away from clean surfaces. Sufficient space must be determined by the initial sizing of the warewash area, as based on the profile or reference size from an existing vessel of the same cruise line per section 6.1.

18.18 Ventilation

For ventilation requirements, see section 14.0.

19.0 Lighting

19.1 Work Surface

Provide a minimum of 220 lux (20 foot-candles) of light at the work surface level in all FOOD PREPARATION, FOOD SERVICE, and warewashing areas when all equipment is installed.

Provide 220 lux (20 foot-candles) of lighting for equipment storage, garbage and food lifts, garbage rooms, and toilet rooms, measured at 760 millimeters (30 inches) above the deck.

19.1.1 Behind and Around Equipment

Provide a minimum light level of 110 lux (10 foot-candles) behind and around equipment as measured at the counter surface or at a distance of 760 millimeters (30 inches) above the deck (e.g., ice machines, combination ovens, beverage dispensers, etc.).

19.1.2 Countertops

Provide a minimum light level of 220 lux (20 foot-candles) at countertops (e.g., beverage lines, etc.).

19.2 Deckhead-mounted Fixtures

For effective illumination, place the deckhead-mounted light fixtures above the work surfaces and position them in an "L" pattern rather than a straight line pattern.

19.3 Installation

Install light fixtures tightly against the bulkhead and deckhead panels. Completely seal electrical penetrations to permit easy cleaning around the fixtures.

19.4 Light Shields

Use shatter-resistant and REMOVABLE light shields for light fixtures. Completely enclose the entire light bulb or fluorescent light tube(s).

19.5 Provision Rooms

Provide lighting levels of at least of 220 lux (20 foot-candles) in provision rooms, measured at 760 millimeters (30 inches) above the deck while the rooms are empty. During normal operations when foods are stored in the rooms, provide lighting levels of at least 110 lux (10 foot-candles), measured at a distance of 760 millimeters (30 inches) above the deck.

19.6 Bars and Waiter Stations

In bars and over dining room waiters' stations designed for lowered lighting during normal operations, provide lighting that can be raised to 220 lux (20 foot-candles) during cleaning operations, as measured at 760 millimeters (30 inches) above the deck. Provide a minimum light level of 110 lux (10 foot-candles) at handwash stations at a bar, and ensure this level is able to be maintained at all times.

19.7 Light Bulbs

Use shielded, coated, or otherwise shatter-resistant light bulbs in areas where there is exposed food; clean equipment, utensils, and linens; or unwrapped single-service and single-use articles. This includes lights above waiter stations.

19.8 Heat Lamps

Use shields that surround and extend beyond bulbs on infrared or other heat lamps to protect against breakage. Allow only the face of the bulb to be exposed.

19.9 Track or Recessed Lights

Decorative track or recessed deckhead-mounted lights above bar countertops, buffets, and other similar areas may be mounted on or recessed within the deckhead panels without being shielded. However, install specially coated, shatter-resistant bulbs in the light fixtures.

20.0 Cleaning Materials, Filters, and Drinking Fountains

20.1 Facilities and Lockers for Cleaning Materials

20.1.1 Racks

Provide bulkhead-mounted racks for brooms and mops or provide sufficient space and hanging brackets within CLEANING LOCKERS. Locate bulkhead-mounted racks outside of FOOD STORAGE, PREPARATION, or SERVICE areas. These racks may be located on the soiled side of warewash areas.

20.1.2 Stainless Steel

Provide stainless steel vented lockers, with COVED junctures, for storing buckets, detergents, sanitizers, cloths, and other wet items.

20.1.3 Size and Location

Size and locate the lockers according to the needs of the vessel and make access convenient.

20.1.3.1 Multiple-level Galleys

If CLEANING LOCKERS are not provided in each of the preparation areas, provide a single CLEANING ROOM for each deck of multiple level galleys. Construct rooms used for cleaning materials in accordance with section 16.0.

20.1.4 Mop Cleaning

Provide facilities equipped with a mop sink and ADEQUATE DECK DRAIN or a pressure washing system for cleaning mops and buckets and that are separate from food facilities. The mop sink may be located on the soiled side of warewash areas.

20.1.5 Labeling

Label all CLEANING LOCKERS and cleaning rooms with the exact wording "CLEANING MATERIALS ONLY."

20.2 Filters

20.2.1 Potable Water Filters

If used, install only point-of-use POTABLE WATER filters on ice machines, combination ovens, beverage machine, etc. Ensure that filters are ACCESSIBLE for changing.

20.3 Drinking Fountains

20.3.1 Outlets Protected

Ensure that the water outlets from drinking fountains are slanted and protected by a sanitary guard.

20.3.2 Food Preparation Areas

Provide drinking fountains with stainless steel cabinets and without filling spouts in FOOD PREPARATION AREAS.

20.3.3 Control

Provide drinking fountains that allow control of the water stream.

20.3.4 Accessible

Install drinking fountains that are ACCESSIBLE to galley personnel.

21.0 Waste Management

21.1 Food and Garbage Lifts

21.1.1 Interiors

Provide food and garbage lifts with interiors that are constructed of stainless steel and meet the same standards as section 16.0.

21.1.2 Decks

Construct decks of a durable, nonabsorbent, NONCORRODING material and with integral COVING.

21.1.3 Air Vents

Position air vents in the upper portion of the bulkhead panels or in the deckhead.

21.1.4 Drain

Install a drain at the bottom of all lift shafts, including provision platform lifts and dumbwaiters.

21.1.5 Dumbwaiter Interiors

Construct the interiors of dumbwaiters of stainless steel with COVED junctures that meet the standards of section 16.0.

21.1.6 Lighting

Provide light fixtures that are recessed or fitted with stainless steel guards.

21.1.7 Garbage Chutes

If installed, construct garbage chutes of stainless steel and with COVED junctures. Install an automatic washing system for the garbage chute. Ensure that the garbage chute meets all SOLAS and classification society requirements.

21.2 Trolley, Waste Container, and Cleaning Equipment Wash Rooms

21.2.1 Construction

Construct bulkheads, deckheads, and decks to the same standards as section 16.0.

21.2.2 Pressure-washing System

Provide a bulkhead-mounted pressure-washing system with a DECK SINK and drain. An enclosed automatic equipment washing machine or room may be used in place of the pressure washing system and DECK SINK.

21.2.3 Handwashing Station

Provide an easily ACCESSIBLE handwashing station that meets the requirements of section 7.1.

21.2.4 Ventilation

Provide ADEQUATE ventilation for the extraction of steam and heat.

21.3 Garbage Holding Facilities

21.3.1 Size and Location

Construct the garbage and refuse storage or holding rooms of sufficient size to hold unprocessed waste for the longest expected time period between off loadings. Separate the refuse-storage room from all FOOD PREPARATION and storage areas.

21.3.2 Ventilation

Provide ADEQUATE supply and exhaust ventilation to control odors, temperature, and humidity. Refer to section 33.0 for other requirements related to ventilation.

21.3.3 Refrigerated Storage

Provide a sealed, refrigerated storage space for wet garbage that meets the requirements of section 15.0.

21.3.4 Handwashing Station

Provide an easily ACCESSIBLE handwashing station that meets the requirements of section 7.1.

21.3.5 Drainage

Provide ADEQUATE deck drainage to prevent pooling of any liquids.

21.3.6 Durable and Easily Cleanable

Ensure that all bulkheads and decks are durable and EASILY CLEANABLE.

21.4 Garbage Processing Areas

21.4.1 Size

Appropriately size the garbage processing area for the operation and supply a sufficient number of sorting tables.

21.4.2 Sorting Tables

Provide stainless steel sorting tables with COVED corners. Provide a table drain and direct it to a strainer-protected DECK DRAIN. If deck coaming is provided, ensure that it is at least 80 millimeters (3 inches) in height and COVED on the inside and outside at the deck juncture.

21.4.3 Handwashing Station

Provide an easily ACCESSIBLE handwashing station that meets the requirements of section 7.1.

21.4.4 Cleaning Locker

Provide a storage locker for cleaning materials that meets the requirements of section 20.1.

21.4.5 Bulkheads and Decks

Ensure that bulkheads and decks are durable, NONCORRODING, and EASILY CLEANABLE.

21.4.5.1 Deck Drains

Provide DECK DRAINS to prevent liquids from pooling on the decks. Provide berm/coaming around all waste-processing equipment and ensure there is ADEQUATE deck drainage inside the berms.

21.4.6 Lighting

Provide light levels of at least 220 lux (20 foot-candles) at the work surface levels and at the handwashing station.

21.4.7 Washing Containers

Equip a sink with a pressure washer or an automatic washing machine for washing garbage/refuse handing equipment, garbage/refuse storage containers, and garbage barrels.

21.5 Black and Gray Water Systems

21.5.1 Drain Lines

Limit the installation of drain lines that carry BLACK WATER or other liquid waste directly overhead or horizontally through spaces used for FOOD AREAS. This includes areas for washing or storage of utensils and equipment, such as in bars and deck pantries and over buffet counters. Sleeve-weld or butt-weld steel pipe and heat fuse or chemically weld plastic pipe.

21.5.1.1 Piping

Do not use push-fit or press-fit piping over these areas. For SCUPPER lines, factory assembled transition fittings for steel to plastic pipes are allowed when manufactured per ASTM F1973 or equivalent standard.

21.5.2 Drainage Systems

Ensure that BLACK and GRAY WATER drainage systems from cabins, FOOD AREAS, and public spaces are designed and installed to prevent waste back up and odor or gas emission into these areas.

21.5.3 Venting

Vent BLACK WATER holding tanks to the outside of the vessel and ensure that vented gases do not enter the vessel through any air intakes.

21.5.4 Independent

Construct BLACK WATER holding tank vents so that they are independent of all other tanks.

21.6 General Hygiene

Construct handwashing stations in the following areas according to section 7.1.

21.6.1 Wastewater Areas

Install at least one handwashing station in each main wastewater treatment, processing, and storage area.

21.6.2 Laundry Areas

Install at least one handwashing station at soiled linen handling areas and at the main exits of the main laundry. Vessel owners will provide locations during the plan review.

21.6.3 Housekeeping Areas

Install handwashing stations in housekeeping areas as described in section 35.1. Provide each handwashing station with a soap dispenser, paper towel dispenser, waste receptacle, and sign that states "wash hands often," "wash hands frequently," or similar wording in English and in other languages, where appropriate.

22.0 Potable Water System

22.1 Striping

22.1.1 Potable Water Lines

Stripe or paint POTABLE WATER lines either in accordance with ISO 14726 (blue/green/blue) or blue only.

22.1.2 Distillate and Permeate Water Lines

Stripe or paint DISTILLATE and PERMEATE WATER LINES directed to the POTABLE WATER system in accordance with ISO 14726 (blue/gray/blue).

22.1.3 Other Piping

No other lines should have the color designations listed in 22.1.1 or 22.1.2.

22.1.4 Intervals

Paint or stripe these lines at 5-meter (15-foot) intervals and on each side of partitions, decks, and bulkheads except where decor would be marred by such markings. This includes POTABLE WATER supply lines in technical lockers.

22.1.5 Downsteam of an RP Assembly

Lines downstream of an RP ASSEMBLY must not be striped as POTABLE WATER.

22.2 Bunker Stations

22.2.1 Position Connections

Position the filling line hose connections at least 450 millimeters (18 inches) above the deck; paint or stripe the filling lines either blue only or in accordance with ISO 14726.

22.2.2 Connection Caps

Equip filling line hose connections with tight-fitting caps that are fastened by a NONCORRODING chain so that the cap does not touch the deck when hanging.

22.2.3 Unique Connections

Use unique connections that only fit POTABLE WATER hoses.

22.2.4 Labeling

Label the filling lines with the exact wording "POTABLE WATER FILLING" with at least 13-millimeter (1/2-inch)-high lettering stamped, stenciled, or painted on the filling lines or on the bulkhead at the filling line.

22.2.5 Filter Location

If any filters are used in the bunkering process, locate them ahead of the halogenation injection point.

Ensure any filters used in the bunkering process are easily ACCESSIBLE and can be removed for inspection and cleaning.

22.3 Filling Hoses

22.3.1 Approved

Provide hoses APPROVED for POTABLE WATER. Hoses must be SMOOTH and durable and have an impervious lining, caps on each end, and fittings unique to the POTABLE WATER connections.

22.3.2 At Least Two Hoses

Provide at least two 15-meter (50-foot) hoses per bunker station.

22.3.3 Label Hoses

Label POTABLE WATER hoses with the exact wording "POTABLE WATER ONLY" with at least 13-millimeter (1/2-inch)-high lettering stamped, stenciled, or painted at each connection end.

22.4 Potable Water Hose Storage

22.4.1 Construction

Construct POTABLE WATER hose lockers from SMOOTH, nontoxic, NONCORRODING, and EASILY CLEANABLE materials.

22.4.2 Mounting

Mount POTABLE WATER hose lockers at least 450 millimeters(18 inches) above the deck.

22.4.3 Self-draining

Design POTABLE WATER hose lockers to be self-draining.

22.4.4 Label Lockers

Label POTABLE WATER hose lockers with the exact wording "POTABLE WATER HOSE AND FITTING STORAGE" in letters at least 13 millimeters (1/2 inch) high.

22.4.5 Size

Provide storage space for at least four 15-meter (50-foot) POTABLE WATER bunker hoses per bunker station.

22.5 International Fire Shore Connections and Fire Sprinkler Shore Connections

22.5.1 RP Assembly

Install an RP ASSEMBLY at all connections where hoses from shore-side POTABLE WATER supplies will be connected to nonpotable systems onboard the vessel.

22.6 Storage and Production Capacity for Potable Water

22.6.1 Minimum Storage Capacity

Provide a minimum of 2 days storage capacity that assumes 120 liters (30 gallons) of water per day per person for the maximum capacity of crew and passengers on the vessel.

22.6.2 Production Capacity

Provide POTABLE WATER production capacity of 120 liters (30 gallons) per day per person for the maximum capacity of crew and passengers on the vessel.

22.7 Potable Water Storage Tanks

22.7.1 General Requirements

22.7.1.1 *Independent of Vessel Shell*

Ensure that POTABLE WATER storage tanks are independent of the shell of the vessel.

22.7.1.2 *No Common Wall*

Ensure that POTABLE WATER storage tanks do not share a common wall with other tanks containing nonpotable water or other liquids.

22.7.1.3 *Cofferdam*

Provide a 450-millimeter (18-inch) cofferdam above and between POTABLE WATER TANKS and tanks that are not for storage of POTABLE WATER and between POTABLE WATER TANKS and the shell. Skin or double-bottom tanks are not allowed for POTABLE WATER storage.

22.7.1.4 *Deck Top*

If the deck is the top of POTABLE WATER TANKS, these tanks must be identified during the plan review. The shipyard will provide the owners a written declaration of the tanks involved and the drawings of the areas that include these tanks.

22.7.1.5 *Tanks with Nonpotable Liquid*

Do not install tanks containing nonpotable liquid directly over POTABLE WATER TANKS.

22.7.1.6 *Coatings*

Use APPROVED POTABLE WATER TANK coatings.

Follow all of the manufacturer's recommendations for applying, drying, and curing the tank coatings.

Provide the following for the tank coatings:
- Written documentation of the approval from the certification organization (independent of the coating manufacturer).
- Manufacturer's recommendations for applying, drying, and curing.

- Written documentation that the manufacturer's recommendations have been followed for applying, drying, and curing.

22.7.1.7 Items That Penetrate Tank
Coat all items that penetrate the tank (e.g., bolts, pipes, pipe flanges) with the same product used for the tank's interior.

22.7.1.8 Super-chlorination
Design tanks to be super-chlorinated one tank at a time.

22.7.1.9 Lines for Nonpotable Liquids
Ensure that lines for nonpotable liquids do not pass through POTABLE WATER TANKS.

22.7.1.10 Nonpotable Lines Above Potable Water Tanks
Minimize the use of nonpotable lines above POTABLE WATER TANKS. If nonpotable water lines are installed, do not use mechanical couplings or push-fit or press-fit piping on lines above tanks. For SCUPPER lines, factory assembled transition fittings for steel to plastic pipes are allowed when manufactured per ASTM F1973 or equivalent standard.

22.7.1.11 Coaming
If coaming is present along the edges or top of the tank, provide slots along the coaming to allow leaking liquids to run off and be detected.

22.7.1.12 Welded Pipes
Treat welded pipes over the POTABLE WATER storage tanks to make them corrosion resistant.

22.7.1.13 Lines Inside Potable Water Tanks
Treat all POTABLE WATER lines inside POTABLE WATER TANKS to make them jointless and NONCORRODING.

22.7.1.14 Label Tanks
Label each POTABLE WATER TANK on its side and where clearly visible, with a number and the exact wording "POTABLE WATER" in letters a minimum of 13 millimeters (1/2 inch) high.

22.7.1.15 Sample Cock
Install at least one sample cock located at least 450 millimeters (18 inches) above the deck plating on each tank. The sample cock must be easily ACCESSIBLE.

Point sample cocks down and identify them with the appropriate tank number.

22.7.2 Storage Tank Access Hatch

22.7.2.1 Installation
Install an access hatch for entry on the sides of POTABLE WATER TANKS.

22.7.3 Storage Tank Water Level

22.7.3.1 Automatic
Provide an automatic method for determining the water level of POTABLE WATER TANKS. Visual sight glasses are acceptable.

22.7.4 Storage Tank Vents

22.7.4.1 Location
Ensure that air-relief vents end at least 1,000 millimeters (40 inches) above the maximum load level of the vessel.

Make the cross-sectional area of the vent equal to or greater than that of the filling line to the tank.

Position the end of the vent so that its opening faces down or is otherwise protected, and install a 16-mesh corrosion-resistant screen.

22.7.4.2 Single Pipe
A single pipe may be used as a combination vent and overflow.

22.7.4.3 Vent Connections
Do not connect the vent of a POTABLE WATER TANK to the vent of a tank that is not a POTABLE WATER TANK.

22.7.5 Storage Tank Drains

22.7.5.1 Design
Design the tanks to drain completely.

22.7.5.2 Drain Opening
Provide a drain opening that is at least 100 millimeters (4 inches) in diameter and preferably matches the diameter of the inlet pipe.

22.7.5.3 Suction Pump
If drained by a suction pump, provide a sump and install the pump suction port in the bottom of the sump.

Install separate pumps and piping not connected to the POTABLE WATER distribution system for draining tanks (Figure 16).

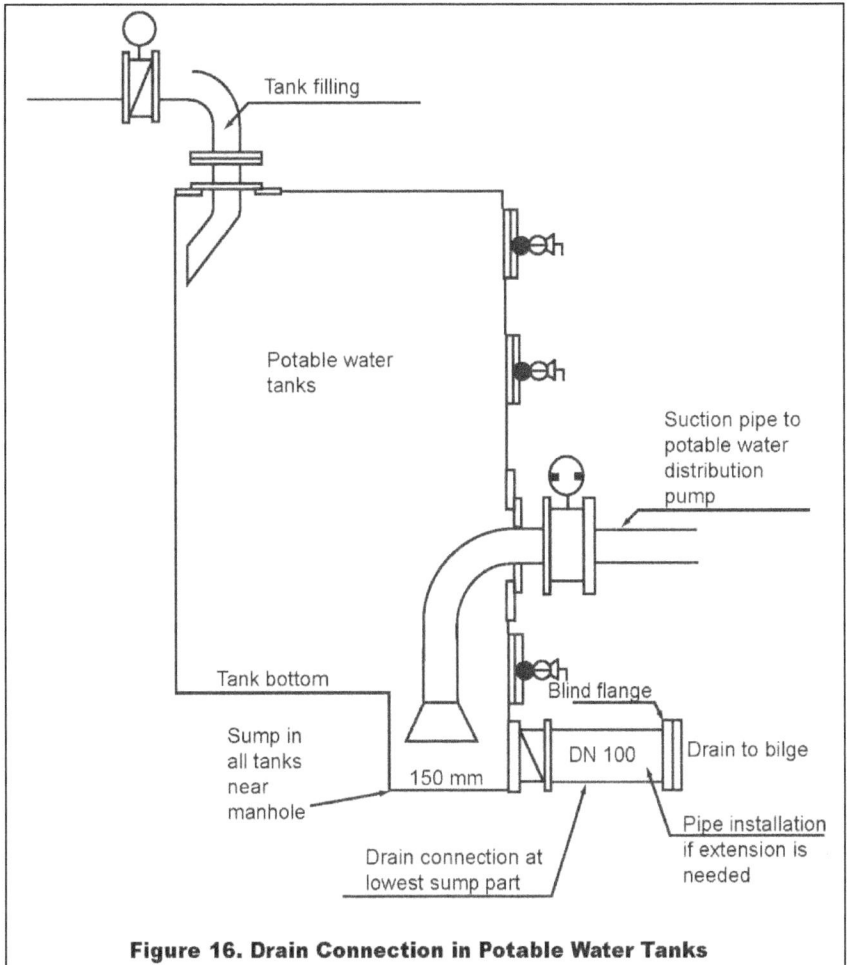

Figure 16. Drain Connection in Potable Water Tanks

22.8   Suction Lines

Place suction lines at least 150 millimeters (6 inches) from the tank bottom or sump bottom.

22.9   Potable Water Distribution System

22.9.1   Location

Locate DISTILLATE, PERMEATE, and distribution lines at least 450 millimeters (18 inches) above the deck plating or the normal bilge water level.

22.9.2   Pipe Materials

Do not use lead, cadmium, or other hazardous materials for pipes, fittings, or solder.

22.9.3   Fixtures That Require Potable Water

Supply only POTABLE WATER to the following areas and plumbing connections, regardless of the locations of these fixtures on the vessel:

- All showers and sinks (not just in cabins).
- Chemical feed tanks for the POTABLE WATER system or RECREATIONAL

WATER systems.

- Drinking fountains.
- Emergency showers.
- Eye wash stations.
- FOOD AREAS.
- Handwash sinks.
- HVAC fan rooms.
- Medical facilities.

Utility sinks for engine/mechanical spaces are excluded.

22.9.4 Paint or Stripe

Paint or stripe POTABLE WATER piping and fittings either blue only or in accordance with ISO 14726 at 5-meter (15-foot) intervals and on each side of partitions, decks, and bulkheads except where the decor would be marred by such markings. This includes POTABLE WATER supply lines in technical lockers.

22.9.5 Steam Generation for Food Areas

Use POTABLE WATER to generate steam applied directly to food and FOOD-CONTACT SURFACES. Generate the steam locally from FOOD SERVICE equipment designed for this purpose (e.g., vegetable steamers, combination-ovens, etc.).

22.9.5.1 Nonpotable Water

Steam generated by nonpotable water may be applied indirectly to food or food equipment if routed through coils, tubes, or separate chambers.

22.10 Disinfection of the Potable Water System

22.10.1 Before Placed in Service

Clean, disinfect, and flush POTABLE WATER TANKS and all parts of the POTABLE WATER system before the system is placed in service.

22.10.2 Free Chlorine Solution

Ensure that DISINFECTION is accomplished by using a 50-MG/L (50-ppm) free chlorine solution for a minimum of 4 hours. Ensure that only POTABLE WATER is used for these procedures. Prior VSP agreement is required if alternative APPROVED DISINFECTION practices are used.

22.10.3 Documentation

Provide written documentation showing that a representative sampling was conducted at various PLUMBING FIXTURES on each deck throughout the vessel (forward, aft, port, and starboard) to ensure that the 50-MG/L (ppm) free chlorine residual has circulated throughout the distribution system to include the distant sampling point(s).

22.11 Potable Water Pressure Tanks

22.11.1 No Connection to Nonpotable Water Tanks

Do not connect POTABLE WATER hydrophore tanks to nonpotable water tanks through the main air compressor.

22.11.2 Filtered Air Supply

Provide a filtered air supply from a dedicated compressor or through a nonpermanent quick disconnect for a PORTABLE compressor. The compressor must not emit oil into the final air product.

22.12 Potable Water Pumps

22.12.1 Size

Size POTABLE WATER pumps to meet the vessel's maximum capacity service demands. Do not use the POTABLE WATER pumps for any other purpose.

22.12.2 Priming

Use nonpriming POTABLE WATER pumps or POTABLE WATER pumps that prime automatically. Use a direct connection when supplying priming water to a POTABLE WATER pump.

22.12.3 Pressure

Properly size POTABLE WATER pumps and distribution lines so that pressure is maintained at all times and at levels to properly operate all equipment.

22.13 Evaporators and Reverse Osmosis Plants

22.13.1 Location of Seawater Inlets

Locate the SANITARY SEAWATER intakes (sea chests) forward of all overboard waste discharge outlets such as emergency and routine discharge lines from waste water treatment facilities, the bilge, RECREATIONAL WATER FACILITIES, and ballast tanks.

This does not include the following:
- Discharges from DECK DRAINS on open decks.
- Cooling lines with no chemical treatment.
- Alarmed vent/overflow pipes for GRAY WATER, treated GRAY or BLACK WATER, and ballast tank with an automatic shutoff system for SANITARY SEAWATER intake. These alarms must be visual and audible and must sound in a space that is continuously occupied.
- Alarmed emergency bilge discharge lines with an automatic shutoff system for SANITARY SEAWATER intake. These alarms must be visual and audible and must sound in a space that is continuously occupied.

22.13.2 Direct Connections

Use only direct connections from the evaporators and reverse osmosis plants to the POTABLE WATER system.

22.13.3 Potable and Nonpotable Water Systems

If an evaporator or reverse osmosis plant makes water for both the POTABLE WATER system and a nonpotable water system, install an AIR GAP or RP ASSEMBLY on the line supplying the nonpotable water system.

22.13.4 Instructions

Post narrative, step-by-step operating instructions for manually operated evaporators and for any reverse osmosis plants near the units.

22.13.5 Discharge to Waste

Ensure that water production units connected to the POTABLE WATER system have the ability to discharge to waste if the distillate is not fit for use.

22.13.6 Indicator and Alarm

Install a low-range salinity indicator, operating temperature indicator, automatic discharge to waste system, and alarm with trip setting on water production equipment.

22.13.7 High-saline Discharge

If routed for discharge, direct high-saline discharge from evaporators to the bilge or overboard through an AIR GAP or RP ASSEMBLY.

22.14 Halogenation

22.14.1 Bunkering and Production

22.14.1.1 Backflow Prevention
Provide POTABLE WATER taps with appropriate BACKFLOW prevention at the HALOGEN supply tanks.

22.14.1.2 Halogen Injection
Control HALOGEN injection by a flow meter or an analyzer with a sample point located at least 3 meters (10 feet) downstream of the HALOGEN injection point. If a static mixer is used in lieu of the 3-meter (10-foot) distance, see section 22.14.2.7 for static mixer requirements.

22.14.1.3 Sample Cock Location
Provide a labeled sample cock at least 3 meters (10 feet) downstream of the HALOGEN injection point.

A static mixer may be used to reduce the distance between the HALOGEN injection point and the sample cock or HALOGEN analyzer sample point. Ensure that the mixer is installed per the manufacturer's recommendation. Provide all manufacturers' literature for installation, operation, and maintenance.

22.14.1.4   pH Adjustment

Provide automatic PH adjustment equipment for water bunkering and production. Install analyzer, controller, and dosing pumps that are designed to accommodate changes in flow rates.

22.14.2   Distribution

22.14.2.1   Sample Point

Provide an analyzer controlled, automatic halogenation system. Install the analyzer probe sample point at least 3 meters (10 feet) downstream of the HALOGEN injection point. If a static mixer is used in lieu of the 3-meter (10-foot) distance, see section 22.14.2.7 for static mixer requirements.

22.14.2.2   Free Halogen Probes

Use probes to measure free HALOGEN and link them to the analyzer/controller and chemical dosing pumps.

22.14.2.3   Backup Halogenation Pump

Provide a back-up halogenation pump with an automatic switchover that begins pumping HALOGEN when the primary (in-use) pump fails or cannot meet the halogenation demand.

22.14.2.4   Probe/Sample Location

Locate HALOGEN analyzer probe and/or sample cock at a distant point in each distribution system loop where significant water flow exists.

22.14.2.5   Alarm

Provide an audible alarm in a continually occupied watch station (e.g., the engine control room or bridge) to indicate low or high free HALOGEN readings at each distant point analyzer.

22.14.2.6   Backflow Prevention

Provide POTABLE WATER taps with appropriate BACKFLOW prevention at HALOGEN supply tanks.

22.14.2.7   Sample Cock Location

Locate a labeled sample cock at least 3 meters (10 feet) downstream of the HALOGEN injection point.

A static mixer may be used to reduce the distance between the HALOGEN injection point and the sample cock or HALOGEN analyzer sample point. Ensure that the mixer is installed per the manufacturer's recommendation. Provide all manufacturers' literature for installation, operation, and maintenance.

22.14.2.8 *Free Halogen Analyzer-chart Recorder*

Provide continuous recording free HALOGEN analyzer-chart recorder(s) that have ranges of 0.0 to 5.0 MG/L (ppm) and indicate the level of free HALOGEN for 24-hour time periods (e.g., circular 24-hour charts).

Electronic data loggers with certified data security features may be installed in lieu of chart recorders. Acceptable data loggers produce records that conform to the principles of operation and data display required of the analog charts, including printing the records. Use electronic data loggers that log times in increments of <15 minutes.

22.14.2.9 *Multiple Distribution Loops*

When supplying POTABLE WATER throughout the distribution network with more than one ring or loop (lower to upper decks or forward to aft), there must be
- Pipe connections that link those loops and a single distant point monitoring analyzer or
- Individual analyzers on each ring or loop.

A single return line that connects to only one ring or loop of a multiple loop system is not acceptable. One chart recorder may be used to record multiple loop readings.

POTABLE WATER distribution loops/rings supplied by separate HALOGEN dosing equipment must include an analyzer chart recorder at a distant point for each loop/ring.

23.0 Cross-connection Control

23.1 Backflow Prevention

Use appropriate BACKFLOW prevention at all CROSS-CONNECTIONS. This may include nonmechanical protection such as an AIR GAP or a mechanical BACKFLOW PREVENTION DEVICE.

23.2 Air Gaps

AIR GAPS should be used where feasible and when water under pressure is not required.

23.3 Atmospheric Vent

A mechanical BACKFLOW PREVENTION DEVICE must have an atmospheric vent.

23.4 Protect Against Health Hazards

Ensure that connections where there is a potential of a health hazard are protected by AIR GAPS or BACKFLOW PREVENTION DEVICES designed to protect against health hazards.

23.5 Test Kit

Provide an appropriate test kit for all testable devices.

Test all testable devices after installation and provide pressure differential test results for each device.

23.6 Atmospheric Vacuum Breaker

When used, install an ATMOSPHERIC VACUUM BREAKER (AVB) 150 millimeters (6 inches) above the fixture flood level rim with no valves downstream of the device.

23.7 Atmospheric or Hose Bib Vacuum Breaker

Ensure an AVB or HOSE-BIB CONNECTED VACUUM BREAKER (HVB) is not installed at a connection where it can be subjected to CONTINUOUS PRESSURE for more than 12 continuous hours.

23.8 Connections Between Potable and Black Water Systems

Ensure that any connection between the POTABLE WATER system and the BLACK WATER system is through an AIR GAP. Where feasible, water required for the BLACK WATER system should not be from the POTABLE WATER system.

23.9 Protection Against Backflow

Protect the following connections to the POTABLE WATER system against BACKFLOW (BACKSIPHONAGE or BACKPRESSURE) with AIR GAPS or mechanical BACKFLOW PREVENTION DEVICES:
- Air conditioning expansion tanks.
- Automatic galley hood washing systems.
- Beauty and barber shop spray-rinse hoses.
- BLACK WATER or combined GRAY WATER/BLACK WATER systems. An AIR GAP is the only allowable protection for these connections.
- Boiler feed water tanks.
- Cabin shower hoses, toilets, WHIRLPOOL SPA tubs, and similar facilities.
- Chemical tanks.
- Decorative water features and fountains.
- Detergent and chemical dispensers.
- Fire system.
- FOOD SERVICE equipment such as coffee machines, ice machines, juice dispensers, combination ovens, and similar equipment.
- Freshwater or saltwater ballast systems.
- Garbage grinders and FOOD WASTE SYSTEMS.
- High saline discharge line from evaporators. An AIR GAP or RP ASSEMBLY are the only allowable protections for these lines.
- Hose-bib connections.
- Hospital and laundry equipment.

- International fire and fire sprinkler water connections. An RP ASSEMBLY is the only allowable device for this connection.
- Mechanical warewashing machines.
- Photographic laboratory developing machines and utility sinks.
- POTABLE WATER, bilge, and sanitary pumps that require priming.
- POTABLE WATER supply to automatic window washing systems that can be used with chemicals or chemical mix tanks.
- RECREATIONAL WATER FACILITIES.
- Spa steam generators where essential oils can be added.
- Toilets, urinals, and shower hoses.
- Water softener and mineralizer drain lines including backwash drain lines. An AG or RP are the only allowable protections for these lines.
- Water softeners for nonpotable fresh water.
- Any other connection between the POTABLE WATER system and a nonpotable water system such as the GRAY WATER, laundry, or TECHNICAL WATER system. An AIR GAP or RP ASSEMBLY are the only allowable forms of protection for these connections.
- Any other connection to the POTABLE WATER system where contamination or BACKFLOW can occur.

23.10   Seawater Lines and Potable Water

Do not make any connections to the SANITARY SEAWATER LINES between the POTABLE WATER production plant supply pump and the POTABLE WATER production plant.

23.11   Seawater Lines and Recreational Water Facilities

Do not make any connections to the SANITARY SEAWATER LINES between the RECREATIONAL WATER FACILITY supply pump and the RWFs.

23.12   Distillate and Permeate Water Lines

Provide an AIR GAP or BACKFLOW PREVENTION DEVICE at connections to the DISTILLATE and PERMEATE WATER LINES intended for the POTABLE WATER system.

23.13   Sanitary Seawater Lines

Provide an AIR GAP or BACKFLOW PREVENTION DEVICE for connections to the SANITARY SEAWATER LINES.

23.14   List of Connections to Potable Water System

A listing must be developed of all connections to the POTABLE WATER system where there is a potential for contamination either with a pollutant or contaminant. At a minimum, this listing must include the following:
- Exact location of the connection.
- PLUMBING FIXTURE (plumbing part [pipe, valve, etc.]) or component connected (what the fixture is connected to [sprinkler, shower, tank, etc.]).
- Form of protection used:

- ○ A<small>IR</small> G<small>APS</small> or
- ○ Manufacturer name and device number (if a device is used).
  - • A testing record for each device with test cocks.

Repeat connections such as toilets and showers can be grouped together under a single listing, as appropriate, with the total number of connections listed.

24.0 Heat Exchangers Used for Cooling or Heating Sanitary Seawater and Potable Water

24.1 Fabrication

Fabricate heat exchangers that use, cool, or heat S<small>ANITARY</small> S<small>EAWATER</small> or P<small>OTABLE</small> W<small>ATER</small> so a single failure of any barrier will not cause a C<small>ROSS-CONNECTION</small> or permit B<small>ACKSIPHONAGE</small> of contaminants into the P<small>OTABLE</small> W<small>ATER</small> system.

24.2 Design

Where both S<small>ANITARY</small> S<small>EAWATER</small> or P<small>OTABLE</small> W<small>ATER</small> and any nonpotable liquid are used, design heat exchangers to protect the S<small>ANITARY</small> S<small>EAWATER</small> or P<small>OTABLE</small> W<small>ATER</small> from contamination by one of the designs in sections 24.2.1 or 24.2.2.

24.2.1 Double-wall Construction

Double-wall construction between the S<small>ANITARY</small> S<small>EAWATER</small> or P<small>OTABLE</small> and nonpotable liquids with both of the following safety features:
- • A void space to allow any leaking liquid to drain away.
- • An alarm system to indicate a leak in the double wall.

24.2.2 Single-wall Construction

Single-wall construction with all of the following safety features:

24.2.2.1 Higher Pressure

Higher pressure of at least 1 bar on the S<small>ANITARY</small> S<small>EAWATER</small> or P<small>OTABLE</small> W<small>ATER</small> side of the heat exchanger.

24.2.2.2 Automatic Valve

An automatic valve arrangement that closes S<small>ANITARY</small> S<small>EAWATER</small> or P<small>OTABLE</small> W<small>ATER</small> circulation in the heat exchanger when the pressure difference is less than 1 bar.

24.2.2.3 Alarm

An alarm system that sounds when the diverter valve directs S<small>ANITARY</small> S<small>EAWATER</small> or P<small>OTABLE</small> W<small>ATER</small> from the heat exchanger.

25.0 Recreational Water Facilities (RWFs) Water Source

25.1 Filling System

Provide a filling system that allows for the filling of each RWF with SANITARY SEAWATER or POTABLE WATER. For a compensation or make-up tank supplied with POTABLE water, an overflow line located below the fill line and at least twice the diameter of the fill line is an acceptable method of BACKFLOW protection provided that the overflow line discharges to the wastewater system through an indirect connection.

25.2 Compensation or Make-up Tank

Where make-up water is required to replace water loss due to splashing, carry out, and other volume loss, install an appropriately designed compensation or make-up tank to ensure that ADEQUATE chemical balance can be maintained.

25.3 Combining RWFs

No more than two similar RWFs may be combined.

CHILDREN'S POOLS and BABY-ONLY WATER FACILITIES must not be combined with any other type of RWFs.

25.4 Independent Manual Testing

When combining RWFs, provisions must be made for independent manual water testing within the mechanical room for each RWF.

25.6 Independent Slide RWF and Adult Swimming Pool

An independent slide RWF and an adult SWIMMING POOL may be combined provided that the water volume added to the slide and the slide pump capacity are sufficient to maintain the TURNOVER rate as shown in section 29.10. Any other combinations of RWFs will be decided on a case-by-case basis during the plan review.

26.0 RWF Showers and Toilet Facilities

26.1 Shower Temperature

Equip showers to provide POTABLE WATER at a temperature not to exceed 43°C (110°F) during normal operations. Install the showers within 10 meters of the entrances to RWFs. The location and number of showers for multifacilities with multiple entrances will be determined during the plan review.

26.2 Showers for Children

RWFs designed for use by children under 6 years of age must have appropriately sized shower facilities. Standard height is acceptable, but the mechanism to operate the flow of water must not be more than 1 meter above the deck.

26.3 Toilet Facilities

Locate toilet facilities within one fire zone (approximately 48 meters [157 feet]) of each RWF and on the same deck. Install a minimum of two separate toilet rooms (either two unisex or one male and one female). Each toilet facility must include a toilet and a handwashing facility. The total number of toilets and toilet facilities required will be assessed during the plan review. Urinals may be installed in addition to the required toilet, but may not replace the toilet.

26.4 Diaper-changing Facilities

Provide diaper changing facilities within one fire zone (approximately 48 meters [157 feet]) and on the same deck of any BABY-ONLY WATER FACILITY. If these facilities are placed within toilet rooms, there must be one facility located within each toilet room (men's, women's, and unisex). Diaper-changing facilities must be equipped in accordance with section 34.2.1.

27.0 RWF Drainage

27.1 Independent System

Provide an independent drainage system for RWFs from other drainage systems. If RWF drains are connected to another drainage system, provide an AIR GAP or a DUAL SWING CHECK VALVE between the two. This includes the drainage for compensation or make-up tanks.

27.2 Slope

Slope the bottom of the RWF toward the drains to achieve complete drainage.

27.3 Seating Drains

If seating is provided inside an RWF, ensure that drains are installed to allow for complete draining of the seating area (including seats inside WHIRLPOOL SPAS and SPA POOLS).

27.4 Drain Completely

Decorative and working features of an RWF must be designed to drain completely and must be constructed of nonporous EASILY CLEANABLE materials. These features must be designed to be shock halogenated.

28.0 RWF Safety

28.1 Antientrapment Drain Covers and Suction Fittings

Where referenced within these guidelines, drain covers must comply with the requirements in ASME A112.19.8-2007, including addenda. See table below for primary and secondary ANTIENTRAPMENT requirements.

VSP is aware that the requirements shown in Table 28.1.7 may not fully meet the letter of the Virginia Graeme Baker Act, but we also recognize the life-safety concerns for rapid dumping of RWFs in conditions of instability at sea. Therefore, it is the owner's decision to meet or exceed VSP requirements.

28.1.1   Installation

Install dual drains that are at least 1 meter (3 feet) apart and at the lowest point in the RWF. Ensure that there are no intermediate drain isolation valves on the lines between the drains (Figure 17a). In a channel system (an UNBLOCKABLE DRAIN), a grate-type cover would be attached to the channel (Figure 17b).

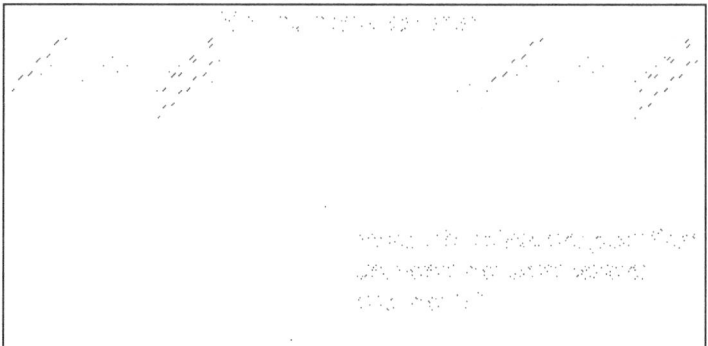

Figure 17a. Dual Drain System

Figure 17b. Channel System

28.1.2   ASME A112.19.8M-2007

When fully assembled and installed, SUCTION FITTINGS must reduce the potential for body entrapment, digit, or limb entrapment in accordance with ASME A112.19.8M-2007.

28.1.3   Stamped and Certified

Manufactured drain covers and SUCTION FITTINGS must be stamped and certified in accordance with the standards set forth in ASME A112.19.8-2007.

28.1.4   Design of Field Fabricated Covers and Fittings

The design of custom/shipyard constructed (field fabricated) drain covers and SUCTION FITTINGS must be fully specified by a registered design professional in accordance with ASME A112.19.8-2007. The specifications must fully address cover/grate loadings; durability; hair, finger, and limb entrapment issues; cover/grate secondary layer of protection; related sump design; and features specific to the RWF.

28.1.5 Alternate to Marking Field Fabricated Fittings

As an alternate to marking custom/shipyard constructed (field fabricated) drain cover fittings, the owner of the facility where these fittings will be installed must be advised in writing by the registered design professional of the information set forth in section 7.1.1 of ASME A112.19.8-2007.

28.1.6 Accompanying Letter

A letter from the shipyard must accompany each custom/shipyard constructed (field fabricated) drain cover fitting. At a minimum, the letter must specify the shipyard, name of the vessel, specifications and dimensions of the drain cover, as noted above, and the exact location of the RWF for which it was designed. The registered design professional's name, contact information, and signature must be on the letter.

28.1.7 Antientrapment/Antientanglement Requirements

See Table 28.1.7 for ANTIENTRAPMENT and ANTIENTANGLEMENT requirements for drains and SUCTION FITTINGS in RWFs.

Table 28.1.7 ANTIENTRAPMENT Requirements for RECREATIONAL WATER FACILITIES
(Does not include facilities designed with zero depth and drains that are not under direct suction)

Option*	Drainage/Recirculation System	Cover Design	Secondary ANTIENTRAPMENT Requirement**
	GRAVITY ONLY		
1	Multiple drains (2 or more drains greater than 1 meter [3 feet] apart)	Standard design (not compliant with ASME A112.19.8)	Alarm
2	Multiple drains (2 or more drains greater than 1 meter [3 feet] apart)	ASME A112.19.8 compliant cover	None
3	Single UNBLOCKABLE DRAIN (per ASME A112.19.8)	Standard design (not compliant with ASME A112.19.8)	Alarm
4	Single UNBLOCKABLE DRAIN (per ASME A112.19.8)	ASME A112.19.8 compliant cover	None
5	Single BLOCKABLE DRAIN or multiple drains (less than 1 meter [3 feet] apart)	ASME A112.19.8 compliant cover	GDS
	SUCTION FITTING		
6	Multiple drains (2 or more drains per pump with drains greater than 1 meter [3 feet] apart)	ASME A112.19.8 compliant cover	None
7	Single UNBLOCKABLE DRAIN (per ASME A112.19.8-2007	ASME A112.19.8 compliant cover	SVRS or APS

| 8 | Single BLOCKABLE DRAIN or multiple drains (less than 1 meter [3 feet] apart) | ASME A112.19.8 compliant cover | SVRS or APS |

*Options 1 through 5 are for fittings that are not under direct suction. These include both fittings to drain the RWF and fittings used to recirculate the water. Options 6 through 8 are for fittings that are under direct suction. These include fittings to drain the RWF and fittings used to recirculate the water.

**Definitions:
- Alarm = the audible alarm must sound in a continuously manned space AND at the RWF. This alarm is for all draining: accidental, routine, and emergency.
- GDS (GRAVITY DRAINAGE SYSTEM) = a drainage system that uses a collector tank from which the pump draws water. Water moves from the RWF to the collector tank due to atmospheric pressure, gravity, and the displacement of water by bathers. There is no direct suction at the RWF.
- SVRS (SAFETY VACUUM RELEASE SYSTEM) = a system that stops the operation of the pump, reverses the circulation flow, or otherwise provides a vacuum release at a suction outlet when a blockage is detected. System must be tested by an independent third party and conform with ASME/ANSI A112.19.17 or ASTM standard F2387.
- APS (AUTOMATIC PUMP SHUT-OFF system) = a device that detects a blockage and shuts off the pump system. A manual shut-off near the RWF does not qualify as an APS.

28.2   Depth Markers

28.2.1   Installation

Install depth markers for each RWF where the maximum water depth is 1 meter (3 feet) or greater. Install depth markers so that they can be seen from the deck and inside the RWF tub. Ensure that the markers are in both meters and feet. Additionally, depth markers must be installed for every 1-meter (3-foot) change in depth.

28.3   Safety Signs

28.3.1   Installation

Install safety signs at each RWF except for BABY-ONLY WATER FACILITIES. At a minimum the signs must include the following words:
- Do not use these facilities if you are experiencing diarrhea, vomiting, or fever.
- No children in diapers or who are not toilet trained.
- Shower before entering the facility.
- Bather load number. (The maximum bather load must be based on the following factor: One person per 19 liters [5 gallons] per minute of recirculation flow.)

Pictograms may replace words, as appropriate or available.

It is advisable to post additional cautions and concerns on signs.

See section 31.3 for safety signs specific to BABY-ONLY WATER FACILITIES and section 32.3 for safety signs specific to WHIRLPOOL SPAS and SPA POOLS.

28.3.1.1   *Children's RWF*

For the children's RWF signs, include the exact wording "TAKE CHILDREN ON FREQUENT BATHROOM BREAKS" or "TAKE CHILDREN ON FREQUENT TOILET BREAKS." This is in addition to the basic RWF safety sign.

28.4   Life-saving Equipment

28.4.1   Location

A rescue or shepherd's hook and an APPROVED floatation device must be provided at a prominent location (visible from the full perimeter of the pool) at each RECREATIONAL WATER FACILITY that has a depth of 1 meter (3 feet) or greater. These devices must be mounted in a manner that allows for easy access during an emergency.

- The pole of the shepherd's hook must be long enough to reach the center of the deepest portion of the pool from the side plus 0.6 meters (2 feet) It must be light, strong, and nontelescoping with rounded nonsharp ends.
- The flotation device must have an attached rope that is at least 2/3 of the maximum pool width.

29.0   Recirculation and Filtration Systems

29.1   Skim Gutters

Where skim gutters are installed, ensure that the maximum fill level of the RWF is to the skim gutter level.

29.2   Overflows

Ensure that overflows are directed by gravity to the compensation or make-up tank for filtration and DISINFECTION. Alternatively, overflows may be directed to the RWF drainage system. If the overflow is connected to another drainage system, provide an AIR GAP or a DUAL SWING CHECK VALVE between the two.

29.3   Return Water

All water returning from an RWF must be directed to the compensation or make-up tank or the filtration and DISINFECTION system.

29.4   Compensation or Make-up Tanks

Ensure that 100% of the water in the compensation or make-up tanks passes through the filtration and DISINFECTION systems before returning to the RWF. This includes any water directed to water features in RWF's.

29.5   Approved

Install recirculation, filtration, and DISINFECTION equipment that has been APPROVED for use in RWFs based on NSF International or an equivalent standard.

29.6   Centrifugal Pumps

Ensure that pumps used to recirculate RWF water are centrifugal pumps that are self-priming or that prime automatically. Flooded end suction pumps are permitted if suitable for the application.

29.7   Skimmers or Gutters

Install surface skimmers or gutters that are capable of handling approximately 80% of the filter flow of the recirculation system.

If skimmers are used instead of gutters, install at least one skimmer for every 37 square meters (400 square feet) of pool surface area.

29.8   Hair and Lint Strainer

Provide a hair and lint strainer between the RWF outlet and the suction side of the pumps to remove foreign debris such as hair, lint, pins, etc.

Ensure that the REMOVABLE portion of the hair and lint strainer is corrosion-resistant and has holes no greater than 6 millimeters (1/4 inch) in diameter.

29.9   Filters

29.9.1   Particle Size

Use filters that are designed to remove all particles greater than 20 microns from the entire volume of the RWF within the specified TURNOVER rate.

29.9.2   Cartridge or Media Type

Use cartridge or media-type filters (e.g., rapid-pressure sand filters, high rate sand filters, diatomaceous earth filters, gravity sand filters). Make filter sizing consistent with American National Standards Institute (ANSI) standards for public RWFs. Ensure that commercial filtration rates for calculations are used for cartridge filters if multiple rates are provided by the manufacturer.

29.9.3   Backwash

Ensure that media-type filters are capable of being backwashed. Provide a clear sight glass on the backwash side of all media filters.

29.9.4   Accessories

Install filter accessories, such as pressure gauges, air-relief valves, and flow meters.

29.9.5   Access

Design and install filters and filter housings in a manner that allows access for inspection, cleaning, and maintenance.

29.9.6   Manufacturer's Information

Provide manufacturer's specifications and recommendations for filtration systems.

29.10   Turnover Rates

Install recirculation pumps, filtration, and DISINFECTION equipment that have the capacity to turn over the RWF water at the appropriate rates as set forth in table the below. Ensure that TURNOVER rates may be increased based on bather load. (The maximum bather load must be based on the following factor: One person per 19 liters [5 gallons] per minute of recirculation flow.)

RECREATIONAL WATER FACILITY	TURNOVER Rate
SWIMMING POOL	4 hours
CHILDREN'S POOL	0.5 hours
WADING POOL	1 hour
WHIRLPOOL SPA	0.5 hours
SPA POOL	2 hours
INTERACTIVE RWF or ACTIVITY POOL (< 610 millimeters [24 inches] deep)	1 hour
INTERACTIVE RWF or ACTIVITY POOL (> 610 millimeters [24 inches] deep)	2 hours
BABY-ONLY WATER FACILITY	0.5 hours
Custom installations (where the above is not applicable)	To be determined by design engineer with VSP review

For a RWF in sea-to-sea mode, ensure a TURNOVER rate of once per hour.

29.11   Primary Disinfection and pH Control

29.11.1   Installation

Install independent automatic analyzer-controlled HALOGEN-based DISINFECTION and pH dosing systems for each RWF or combined RWFs as allowed in sections 25.3 and 25.6. The analyzer must be capable of measuring HALOGEN levels in MG/L (ppm) and pH levels. Analyzers must have digital readouts that indicate measurements from the installed analyzer probes.

29.11.2   Monitoring and Recording

Provide an automatic monitoring and recording system for the free HALOGEN residuals in MG/L (ppm) and pH levels. The recording system must be capable of recording these levels 24 hours/day.

Install chart recorders or electronic data loggers with security features that record pH and HALOGEN measurements.

Electronic data loggers must be capable of recording in increments of ≤ 15 minutes.

The probe for the automated analyzer recorder must be installed before the compensation or make-up tank or from a line taken directly from the RWF.

Install appropriate sample taps for analyzer calibration.

29.11.3 Analyzer Probes

For WHIRLPOOL SPAS and SPA POOLS, analyzer probes for the dosing and recording system must be capable of measuring and recording levels up to 10 MG/L (10 ppm).

29.11.4 Alarm

Provide an audible alarm in a continuously occupied watch station (e.g., the engine control room) to indicate low and high free HALOGEN and pH readings in each RWF.

29.11.5 Water Feature Design

Design water features such that the water cannot be taken directly from the compensation or make-up tank but must be first routed through filtration and DISINFECTION systems.

29.11.6 Water Supply

Water may be taken directly from the RWF to supply other features within the same RWF. If taken from the RWF, consider taking the water from the lower part of the RWF. This does not apply to a BABY-ONLY WATER FACILITY.

29.12 Secondary Disinfection

29.12.1 Installation

Install a secondary DISINFECTION system for each CHILDREN'S POOL, INTERACTIVE RECREATIONAL WATER FACILITIES, and BABY-ONLY WATER FACILITY.

29.13 RWF Mechanical Room (Pump Room)

29.13.1 Accessible

Make RWF mechanical rooms ACCESSIBLE and well-ventilated.

29.13.2 Design

Design pump rooms so that operators are not required to stoop, bend, or crawl and can easily access and perform routine maintenance and duties.

29.13.3 Clearance

Provide sufficient clearance between the top of components such as compensation or make-up tanks and filter housings and the deckhead for inspection, maintenance, and cleaning. This could be accomplished by providing a hatch in the deckhead above.

29.13.4 Mark Piping

Mark all piping with directional-flow arrows and provide a flow diagram and operational instructions for each RWF in a readily available location.

29.13.5 Chemical Storage and Refill

Design the RWF mechanical room for safe chemical storage and refilling of chemical feed tanks.

29.13.6 Deck Drains

Install DECK DRAINS in each RWF mechanical room that allow for draining of the entire pump, filter system, compensation or make-up tank, and associated piping. Provide sufficient drainage to prevent pooling on the deck.

29.14 RWF System Drainage

29.14.1 Installation

Install drains in the RWF system to allow for complete drainage of the entire volume of water from the pump, filter system, compensation or make-up tank, and all associated piping.

29.14.2 Compensation Tank Drain

Provide a drain at the bottom of each compensation or make-up tank to allow for complete draining of the tank. Install an access port for cleaning the tank and for the addition of batch halogenation and pH control chemicals.

29.14.3 Utility Sink

Install a utility sink and a hose-bib tap supplied with POTABLE WATER in each RWF pump room. A threaded hose attachment at the utility sink is acceptable for the tap.

30.0 Additional Requirements for Children's Pools

30.1 Prevent Access

Provide a method to prevent access to pools located in remote areas of the vessel.

30.2 Design

Design the pool such that the maximum water level cannot exceed 1 meter (3 feet).

30.3 Secondary Disinfection System

30.3.1 Secondary UV Disinfection

In addition to the HALOGEN DISINFECTION system, provide a secondary UV

DISINFECTION system capable of inactivating *Cryptosporidium*. Ensure that these systems are installed in accordance with the manufacturer's specifications. Secondary UV DISINFECTION systems must be designed to operate in accordance with the parameters set forth in NSF International or equivalent standard.

30.3.2 Sized

Secondary DISINFECTION systems must be appropriately sized to disinfect 100% of the water at the appropriate TURNOVER rate. Secondary DISINFECTION systems are to be installed after filtration but before HALOGEN-based DISINFECTION. Unless otherwise accepted by the VSP, secondary DISINFECTION must be accomplished by a UV DISINFECTION system.

30.3.3 Low- and Medium-pressure UV Systems

Low- and medium-pressure UV systems can be used and must be designed to treat 100% of the flow through the feature line(s). Multiple units are acceptable. UV systems must be designed to provide 40 mJ/cm^2 at the end of lamp life. UV systems must be rated at a minimum of 254 nm.

30.3.4 Cleaning

Install UV systems that allow for cleaning of the lamp jacket without dissembling the unit.

30.3.5 Spare Lamp

A spare ultraviolet lamp must and any accessories required by the manufacturer to change the lamp must be provided. Additionally, operational instructions for the UV DISINFECTION system must be provided.

31.0 Additional Requirements for Baby-only Water Facility
The operational requirements for this RWF will be through a variance only.

31.1 Water Source

31.1.1 Compensation or Makeup Tank
Fill water must be provided only to the compensation or make-up tank and not directly to the SPRAY PAD.

31.2 Baby-only Water Facility

31.2.1 Deck Material
Ensure that the decking material for the facility is durable, nonabsorbent, slip-resistant, and nontoxic. If climbing features are installed, provide impact attenuation surfaces in accordance with ASTM F1292-04.

31.2.2 Limit Access
If located near other RWFs, design the facility to limit access to and from

surrounding RWFs.

31.2.3   Deck Surface

Design and slope the deck surface of the BABY-ONLY WATER FACILITY to ensure complete drainage and prevent pooling/ponding of water (zero depth).

31.2.4   Gravity Drains

Provide ADEQUATE GRAVITY DRAINS throughout the SPRAY PAD to allow for complete drainage of SPRAY PAD. Suction drains are not permitted.

31.2.5   Filtration and Disinfection

Ensure that 100% of the GRAVITY DRAINS are directed to the BABY-ONLY WATER FACILITY compensation or make-up tank for filtration and DISINFECTION before return to the SPRAY PAD.

31.2.6   Divert Water to Waste

Provide a means to divert water from the SPRAY PAD to waste. If the water from the pad is directed to the wastewater system, ensure there is an indirect connection such as an AIR GAP or AIR-BREAK.

31.2.7   Prevent Water Runoff

Any spray features must be designed and constructed to prevent water run-off from the surrounding deck from entering the BABY-ONLY WATER FACILITY.

31.3   Safety Sign

31.3.1   Content

Install an easy-to-read permanent sign, with letters at least 25 millimeters (1 inch) high, at each entrance to the BABY-ONLY WATER FACILITY feature. At a minimum, the sign should state the following:
- This facility is intended for use by children in diapers or children who are not completely toilet trained.
- Use of this facility may put children at increased risk for illness.
- Children who have a medical condition that may put them at increased risk for illness should not use these facilities.
- Children who are experiencing symptoms such as vomiting, diarrhea, skin sores, or infections are prohibited from using these facilities.
- Children must wear a swim diaper.
- Children must be accompanied by an adult at all times.
- Ensure that children have a clean swim diaper before using these facilities. Frequent swim diaper changes are recommended.
- Do not change diapers in the area of the BABY-ONLY WATER FACILITY. A diaper changing station has been provided (give exact location) for your convenience.

31.4 Recirculation and Filtration System

31.4.1 Compensation or Makeup Tank

Install a compensation or make-up tank with an automatic level control system capable of holding an amount of water sufficient to ensure continuous operation of the filtration and DISINFECTION systems. This capacity must be equal to at least 3 times the total operating volume of the system.

31.4.2 Accessible Drain

Install an ACCESSIBLE drain at the bottom of the tank to allow for complete draining of the tank. Install an access port for cleaning the tank and for the addition of batch halogenation and pH control chemicals.

31.4.3 Secondary Disinfection and pH Systems

Design the system so that 100% of the water for the BABY-ONLY WATER FACILITY feature passes through filtration, halogenation, secondary DISINFECTION, and pH systems before returning to the BABY-ONLY WATER FACILITY.

31.5 Disinfection and pH Control

31.5.1 Independent Automatic Analyzer

Install independent automatic analyzer-controlled HALOGEN-based DISINFECTION and pH dosing systems. The analyzer must be capable of measuring HALOGEN levels in MG/L (ppm) and pH levels. Analyzers must have digital readouts that indicate measurements from the installed analyzer probes.

31.5.2 Automatic Monitoring and Recording

Provide an automatic monitoring and recording system for the free HALOGEN residuals in MG/L (ppm) and pH levels. The recording system must be capable of recording these levels 24 hours/day.

31.5.3 Secondary Disinfection System

31.5.3.1 *Cryptosporidium*

Provide a secondary UV DISINFECTION system capable of inactivating *Cryptosporidium*. Ensure that these systems are installed in accordance with the manufacturer's specifications. Secondary UV DISINFECTION systems must be designed to operate in accordance with the parameters set forth in NSF International for use in BABY-ONLY WATER FACILITIES.

31.5.3.2 *Size*

Secondary DISINFECTION systems must be appropriately sized to disinfect 100% of the water at the appropriate TURNOVER rate. Secondary DISINFECTION systems are to be installed after filtration but before HALOGEN-based DISINFECTION. Unless otherwise APPROVED by

VSP, secondary DISINFECTION must be accomplished by a UV DISINFECTION system.

31.5.3.3 Low- and Medium-pressure UV Systems
Low- and medium-pressure UV systems can be used and must be designed to treat 100% of the flow through the feature line(s). Multiple units are acceptable. UV systems must be rated at a minimum of 254 nm. UV systems must be designed to provide 40 mJ/cm^2 at the end of lamp life.

31.5.3.4 Cleaning
Install UV systems that allow for cleaning of the lamp jacket without dissembling the unit.

31.5.3.5 Spare Lamp
A spare ultraviolet lamp and any accessories required by the manufacturer to change the lamp must be provided. In addition, operational instructions for the UV DISINFECTION system must be provided.

31.6 Automatic Shut-off

31.6.1 Installation
Install an automatic control that shuts off the water supply to the BABY-ONLY WATER FACILITY if the free HALOGEN residual or pH range have not been met per the requirements set forth in the current *VSP 2011 Operations Manual*. The shut-off control must operate similarly when the UV DISINFECTION system is not operating within acceptable parameters.

31.7 Baby-only Water Facility Pump Room

31.7.1 Discharge
All recirculated water discharged to waste must be through a visible indirect connection in the pump room.

31.7.2 Flow Meter
A flow meter must be installed in the return line before HALOGEN injection. The flow meter must be accurate to within 10% of actual flow.

32.0 Additional Requirements for Whirlpool Spas and Spa Pools
WHIRLPOOL SPAS that are similar in design and construction to public WHIRLPOOL SPAS but which are located for the sole use of an individual cabin or groups of cabins must comply with the public WHIRLPOOL SPA requirements if the WHIRLPOOL SPA has either of the following features:
- Tub capacity of more than four individuals.
- Location outside of cabin or cabin balcony.

32.1 Overflow System

For WHIRLPOOL SPAS, design the overflow system so the water level is maintained.

32.2 Temperature Control

Provide a temperature control mechanism to prevent the temperature from exceeding 40°C (104°F).

32.3 Safety Sign

In addition to the RWF safety sign in section 28.3, install a sign at each WHIRLPOOL SPA and SPA POOL entrance listing precautions and risks associated with the use of these facilities. At a minimum, include a caution against use by the following:
- Individuals who are immunocompromised.
- Individuals on medication or who have underlying medical conditions, such as cardiovascular disease, diabetes, or high or low blood pressure.
- Children, pregnant women, and elderly persons.

Additionally, caution against exceeding 15 minutes of use.

32.4 Drainage System

For WHIRLPOOL SPAS, provide a line in the drainage system to allow these facilities to be drained to the GRAY WATER, TECHNICAL WATER, or other wastewater holding system through an indirect connection or a DUAL SWING CHECK VALVE. This does not include the BLACK WATER system.

33.0 Ventilation Systems

33.1 Air Supply Systems

33.1.1 Accessible

Design and install air handling units to be ACCESSIBLE for periodic inspections and air intake filter changing.

33.1.2 Drain Completely

Install air condition condensate collection pans that drain completely.

Connect condensate collection pans to drain piping to prevent condensate from pooling on the decks.

33.1.3 Air Intakes

Locate air intakes for fan rooms so that any ventilation or processed exhaust air is not drawn back into the vessel.

33.1.4 Makeup Air Supply

Provide a sufficient make-up air supply in all FOOD PREPARATION, warewashing, CLEANING, and toilet rooms.

33.1.5 Air Vent Diffusers

Design all cabin air vent diffusers to be REMOVABLE.

33.1.6 Condensate Collection Pans

Make air handling unit condensate collection pans READILY ACCESSIBLE for inspection, cleaning, and maintenance. Provide access panels to all major air supply trunks to allow periodic inspection and cleaning.

33.1.7 Engine Room and Mechanical Spaces

Provide a separate independent air supply system for the engine room and other mechanical spaces (e.g., fuel separation, purifying, and BLACK WATER treatment rooms).

33.2 Air Exhaust Systems

33.2.1 Independent Systems

Air handling units in the areas noted in sections 33.2.1.1 through 33.2.1.6 must exhaust air through independent systems that are completely separated from systems using recirculated air.

33.2.1.1 Engine Rooms and Mechanical Spaces
Engine rooms and other mechanical spaces;

33.2.1.2 Medical or Isolation Spaces
Hospitals, infirmaries, and any rooms designed for patient care or isolation.

33.2.1.3 RWFs
Indoor RECREATIONAL WATER FACILITIES, dome-type RECREATIONAL WATER FACILITIES when closed, and supporting mechanical rooms.

33.2.1.4 Galleys
Galleys and other FOOD PREPARATION AREAS.

33.2.1.5 Toilet
Cabin and public toilet rooms.

33.2.1.6 Waste Processing Areas
Waste processing areas.

33.2.2 Negative Air Pressure

Maintain negative air pressure, in relation to the surrounding areas, in the areas listed in sections 33.2.1.1 through 33.2.1.6.

33.2.3 Sufficient Exhaust

Provide a sufficient exhaust system in all FOOD PREPARATION, warewashing, CLEANING, and toilet rooms to keep them free of excessive heat, humidity, steam, condensation, vapors, obnoxious odors, and smoke.

33.2.4　Access Panels

Provide access panels to all major air exhaust trunks to allow periodic inspection and cleaning.

33.2.5　Written Balancing Report

Provide a written ventilation system balancing report for areas listed in sections 33.2.1.1 through 33.2.1.6.

34.0　Child Activity Center

34.1　Facilities

Include the following in CHILD ACTIVITY CENTER (this does not apply for areas only for children 6 years of age and older).

34.1.1　Handwashing

Handwashing facilities must be provided in each CHILD ACTIVITY CENTER. They must be ACCESSIBLE to each CHILD ACTIVITY CENTER without barriers such as doors. Locate the handwashing facility outside of the toilet room and install handwashing sinks with a maximum height of 560 millimeters (22 inches) above the deck.

- Provide hot and cold POTABLE WATER to all handwashing sinks.
- Equip handwashing sinks to provide water at a temperature not to exceed 43°C (110°F) during use.
- Provide handwashing facilities that include a soap dispenser, paper towel dispenser or air dryer, and a waste receptacle.

34.1.2　Toilet Rooms

Toilet rooms must be provided in CHILD ACTIVITY CENTERS. Provide one toilet for every 25 children or fraction thereof, based on the maximum capacity of the center. The toilet rooms must include items noted in sections 34.1.2.1 through 34.1.2.6.

34.1.2.1　Child-sized Toilets

CHILD-SIZED TOILETS with a maximum height of 280 millimeters (11 inches) (including the toilet seat) and toilet seat opening no greater than 203 millimeters (8 inches).

34.1.2.2　Handwashing Facilities

- Provide hot and cold POTABLE WATER to all handwashing sinks.
- Equip handwashing sinks to provide water at a temperature not to exceed 43°C (110°F) during use.
- Install handwashing sinks with a maximum height of 560 millimeters (22 inches) above the deck.
- Provide handwashing facilities that include a soap dispenser and paper towel dispenser or air dryer, and a waste receptacle.

34.1.2.3   *Storage*
Provide storage for gloves and wipes.

34.1.2.4   *Waste Receptacle*
Provide an airtight, washable, waste receptacle.

34.1.2.5   *Self-closing Doors*
Provide self-closing toilet room exit doors.

34.1.2.6   *Sign*
Provide a sign with the exact wording "WASH YOUR HANDS AND ASSIST THE CHILDREN WITH HANDWASHING AFTER HELPING THEM USE THE TOILET." The sign should be in English and can also be in other languages.

34.2   Diaper-changing Station
Provide a diaper-changing station in CHILD ACTIVITY CENTERS where children in diapers or children who are not toilet trained will be accepted.

34.2.1   Supplies
Include the following in each diaper changing station:
- A diaper-changing table that is impervious, nonabsorbent, nontoxic, SMOOTH, durable, and cleanable, and designed for diaper changing.
- An airtight, soiled-diaper receptacle.
- An adjacent handwashing station equipped in accordance with section 34.1.2.2.
- A storage area for diapers, gloves, wipes, and disinfectant.
- A sign stating with the exact wording "WASH YOUR HANDS AFTER EACH DIAPER CHANGE." The sign should be in English and can also be in other languages.

34.3   Child-care Providers
Provide toilet and handwashing facilities for child care providers that are separate from the children's toilet rooms. A public toilet outside the center is acceptable.

34.4   Furnishings
Surfaces of tables, chairs, and other furnishings must be constructed of an EASILY CLEANABLE, nonabsorbent material.

35.0   Housekeeping

35.1   Handwashing Stations
Provide handwashing stations for housekeeping staff. VSP will evaluate the number and location for these handwashing stations during the plan review process.

35.1.1 Location

Ensure that at least one handwashing station is available for each cabin attendant work zone and on the same deck as the work zone. One handwashing station may be located between two cabin attendant work zones, and travel across crew passageways is permitted.

35.1.2 Ice/Deck Pantries

Handwashing stations for housekeeping staff include those in ice/deck pantries, but do not include those located in bars, room service pantries, bell boxes, or other FOOD AREAS.

35.1.3 Supplies

Handwashing stations not located in ice/deck pantries must have a paper towel dispenser, soap dispenser, and a waste receptacle. These stations must provide water at a temperature between 38°C (100°F) and 49°C (120°F) through a mixing valve and be installed to allow for easy access by cabin attendants. Handwash stations inside of ice/deck pantries must be installed in accordance with section 7.1.

36.0 Passenger and Crew Public Toilet Rooms

36.1 No-touch Exits

Provide either of the following in the public toilet rooms:

36.1.1 Hands-free Exit

Hands-free exits from toilet rooms (such as doorless entry, automatic door openers, latchless doors that open out), or

36.1.2 Paper Towel Dispensers and Waste Receptacle

Paper towel dispensers at or after handwashing stations and a waste receptacle near the last exit door(s) to allow for towel disposal.

36.2 Self-closing Doors

All public toilet room exit doors must be self-closing.

37.0 Decorative Fountains and Misting Systems

37.1 Potable Water

Provide POTABLE WATER to all decorative fountains, misting systems, and similar facilities.

37.2 Design

Design and install decorative fountains, misting systems and similar facilities to be maintained free of *Mycobacterium*, *Legionella*, algae, and mold growth.

37.3 Automated Treatment

Install an automated treatment system (halogenation, UV, or other effective disinfectant) to prevent the growth of *Mycobacterium* and *Legionella* in any recirculated decorative fountain, misting system, or similar facility. Ensure that these systems can also be manually disinfected.

37.4 Manual Disinfection

Provide a plumbing connection for manual disinfection for all non-recirculated decorative fountains, misting systems, or similar facilities.

37.5 Water Temperature

If heat is used as a disinfectant, ensure that the water temperature, as measured at the misting nozzle, can be maintained at 65°C (149°F) for a minimum of 10 minutes.

37.6 Removable Nozzles

Ensure that misting nozzles are REMOVABLE for cleaning and DISINFECTION.

37.7 Schematics

Provide operational schematics for misting systems.

38.0 Acknowledgments

38.1 Individuals

This document is a result of the cooperative effort of many individuals from the government, private industry, and the public. VSP thanks all of those who submitted comments and participated throughout this lengthy process.

38.2 Standards, Codes, and Other References Reviewed for Guidance

American National Standards Institute/National Spa & Pool Institute. 2004. NSF/ANSI 50-2004. Standard for public swimming pools and standard for public spas, standard 50: circulation system components and related materials for swimming pools, spas/hot tubs. Ann Arbor, MI: NSF International. http://www.nsf.org/.

American National Standards Institute/The Association of Pool & Spa Professionals. 2006. ANSI/APSP-7 2006. American National Standard for suction entrapment avoidance in swimming pools, wading pools, spas, hot tubs, and catch basins. Alexandria, VA: The Association of Pool & Spa Professionals. http://www.apsp.org.

American Society of Heating, Refrigerating, and Air-Conditioning Engineers. 2000. ASHRAE Standard 12-2000. Minimizing the risk of Legionellosis associated with building water systems. Atlanta, GA: American Society of Heating, Refrigerating, and Air-Conditioning Engineers. http://www.ashrae.org/.

American Society of Sanitary Engineering. 2008. ANSI/ASSE #1001 - 2008, Atmospheric type vacuum breakers. Westlake, OH. American Society of Sanitary Engineering.

American Academy of Pediatrics, American Public Health Association, and National Resource Center for Health and Safety in Child Care and Early Education. 2002. Caring for our children: national health and safety performance standards; guidelines for out-of-home child care programs, 2nd edition. Elk Grove Village, IL: American Academy of Pediatrics and Washington, DC: American Public Health Association; 238. Available from URL: http://nrckids.org/CFOC/.

Centers for Disease Control and Prevention. 1997. Final recommendations to minimize transmission of Legionnaires' disease from whirlpool spas on cruise ships. Atlanta: U.S. Department of Health and Human Services.

Centers for Disease Control and Prevention. 2000, 2005. Vessel Sanitation Program 2000 operations manual. Atlanta: U.S. Department of Health and Human Services. Available from URL: http://www.cdc.gov/nceh/vsp/pub/pub.htm.

Food and Drug Administration. 1997, 1999, 2001, 2005, 2009. Food code. Rockville, MD: U.S. Department of Health and Human Services. Available from URL: http://www.fda.gov/Food/FoodSafety/RetailFoodProtection/FoodCode/default.htm.

Food and Drug Administration. 2000. Food Establishment Plan Review Guide. Rockville, MD: U.S. Department of Health and Human Services. Available from URL: http://www.fda.gov/Food/FoodSafety/RetailFoodProtection/ComplianceEnforceme nt/ucm101639.htm.

Foundation for Cross-Connection Control and Hydraulic Research. Manual of cross-connection control, 10th edition. Los Angeles, CA: University of Southern California.

International Association of Plumbing and Mechanical Officials. 2003. Uniform plumbing code. Uniform Plumbing Code-IAPMO/ANSI UPC 1-2003. Ontario, CA: International Association of Plumbing and Mechanical Officials. Available from URL: http://iapmostore.org/.

International Code Council. 2003. International electric code. Washington, DC: International Code Council. Available from URL: http://www.iccsafe.org/.

International Maritime Organization. 2009. International Convention for the Safety of Life at Sea (SOLAS), 1974, as amended; consolidated edition. London, UK: International Maritime Organization.

International Organization for Standardization. 2002. Ships and marine technology – identification colours for the content of piping systems, ISO 14726-2. Geneva: International Organization for Standardization. Available from URL: http://www.iso.org/iso/catalogue_detail.htm?csnumber=28353.

National Resource Center for Health and Safety in Child Care and Early Education. http://nrckids.org/.

National Swimming Pool Foundation. 2007. Certified Pool-Spa Operator Handbook, 2007 Edition. For more information, visit URL: http://www.nspf.org.

NSF International. 2005. Certification policies for food equipment and ANSI/NSF International Standards 2–59 for food equipment, through 2005. Ann Arbor, MI: NSF International. Available from URL: http://www.nsf.org/Certified/Food/.

Plumbing-Heating-Cooling Contractors Association. 2003. National Standard Plumbing Code with illustrations. Falls Church, VA: Plumbing-Heating-Cooling Contractors Association. Available from URL: http://www.phccweb.org/.

Underwriters Laboratories. For information on UL standards, visit URL: http://www.ul.com/global/eng/pages/offerings/services/productsafety/.

U.S. Consumer Product Safety Commission. 2010. Pool and spa safety. Bethesda, MD: U.S. Consumer Product Safety Commission. Available from URL: http://www.poolsafely.gov/pool-spa-safety/.

World Health Organization. 2011. Guide to ship sanitation. 3rd edition. Geneva: World Health Organization. Available from URL: http://apps.who.int/bookorders/anglais/detart1.jsp?sesslan=1&codlan=1&codcol=15&codcch=3055.

World Health Organization. 2008. Guidelines for drinking water quality. 3rd edition. Geneva: World Health Organization. Available from URL: http://www.who.int/water_sanitation_health/dwq/guidelines/en/.

39.0 Appendices

39.1 Sample Letter of Request for Construction Inspection

(Company or Organization Letterhead)
Chief, Vessel Sanitation Program
National Center for Environmental Health
Centers for Disease Control and Prevention (CDC)
4770 Buford Highway, NE, MS F-59
Atlanta, GA 30341-3717

Fax: 770-488-4127

We request the presence of USPHS representatives to conduct a construction inspection on the cruise vessel (NAME). We tentatively expect to deliver the vessel on (DATE). We would like to schedule the inspection for (DATE) in (CITY, COUNTRY). We expect the inspection to take approximately (NUMBER OF DAYS). We will pay CDC in accordance with the inspection fees published in the *Federal Register*.

For inspections occurring outside of the United States, we will make all necessary arrangements for lodging and transportation of the Vessel Sanitation Program staff conducting this inspection, which includes airfare and ground transportation in (CITY, COUNTRY). We will provide in-kind lodging, airfare, and local transportation expenses from (U.S. DEPARTURE DATE) to (U.S. RETURN DATE). No cash or honorarium will be given. No U.S. federal funds will be used.

Send invoice to:

Company (note: if a U.S. company, provide your federal tax identification number)
Attention:
Street Address
City, State, Country
Zip Code
Office Telephone Number
Office Fax Number

If you have any questions concerning this request, please contact:
(Signed)
Name and Title

Note: this letter must be signed and on company/organization letterhead

39.2   VSP Contact Information

39.2.1   Atlanta Office

CDC/NCEH/Vessel Sanitation Program
4770 Buford Highway, NE/MS F-59
Atlanta, GA 30341-3724
Phone: 770-488-7070
Fax: 770-488-4127
E-mail: vsp@cdc.gov

39.2.2   Fort Lauderdale Office

CDC/NCEH/Vessel Sanitation Program
1850 Eller Drive, Suite 101
Ft Lauderdale, FL 33316-4201
Phone: 1-800-323-2132 or 954-356-6650

Fax: 954-356-6671

39.2.3 VSP Web Site

For updates to these guidelines and information about the Vessel Sanitation Program, visit http://www.cdc.gov/nceh/vsp.

39.3 VSP Construction Checklists

39.3.1 Available

VSP developed checklists from these guidelines that may be helpful to shipyard and cruise industry personnel in achieving compliance with these guidelines. Contact VSP for a copy of these checklists.

40.0 Vessel Profile Worksheet

Vessel Name: Date:

FOOD SERVICE AREAS

Description	Number	Location (Deck #)
Galley		
Main		
Buffet		
Crew		
Other		
Bars		
Pantries		
Bar		
Deck		
Ice		
Room Service		
Bell Box		
Provisions		
Preparation		
Rooms		
Vegetable		
Butcher		
Fish		
Bakery		
Fruit		
Buffet		
Buffets		
Passenger		
Crew		
Staff		
Officer		
Others		
Pizzeria		
Sushi		

Description	Number	Location (Deck #)
Others (con't.)		
Grill		
Ice Cream		
Specialty		

POTABLE WATER

Description	Number	Location (Deck #)
Bunker		
Stations		
Filters		
Chlorinators		
Analyzer/Recorder		
pH Control		
Production		
Evaporator		
Osmosis		
Chlorinator		
Analyzer/Recorder		
Storage		
Potable Tanks		
Skin/Double		
Bottoms		
Manual Sounding		

BACKFLOW Protection

Location	Type	Filled By
Technical Tanks		
Laundry Tanks		
Boiler Feed Tanks		
Distribution		
Analyzer/Recorder		
Point Source		
Filters		

Key

Filled by
Bunker   B
Evaporator/RO   E/O
Potable Water   PW
Condensate   C
Technical   T
Other   Oth

Type
Air Gap   AG
Reduced Pressure Principle   RP
Atmospheric Vacuum Breaker   AVB
Continuous Pressure   CP

Vessel Name:

Date:

Gross Registered Tonnage:

Max Passengers:

Max Crew:

BACKFLOW Protection

System	Type	Location (Deck #)
A/C Expansion Tank		
Beauty Salon		
Deckwashing Taps		
Fuel Oil Separator		
Lube Oil Separator		
Hood Cleaning		
Hospital		
Hydrophore Tank		
International Shore Con.		
Laundry (Main)		
Launderettes		
Photo Lab		
Toilets		
Multiflow		
Pulper System		
Showers		
Steam Generators (Spas)		
WHIRLPOOL SPAS		
SWIMMING POOLS		
Sprinkler System		
High Saline Discharge (Evap)		
Mineralizer		
Garbage Room		
Others		

Key

Type of BACKFLOW Preventer

AIR GAP	AG
REDUCED PRESSURE PRINCIPLE	RP
ATMOSPHERIC VACUUM BREAKER	AVB
CONTINUOUS PRESSURE Type	CP
Noncontinuous Pressure Type	NCP
None Required	NR

Recreational Waters
SWIMMING POOLS

Fresh Water Pools	No.	Location (Deck #)
Halogenation	Y/N	
Chlorine		
Bromine		
Recorder		

Seawater Pools

Flow Through	No.	Location (Deck #)
Recirculation		
Halogenation	Y/N	
Chlorine		
Bromine		
Recorder		

Fresh/Seawater Pools

Flow Through	No.	Location (Deck #)
Recirculation		
Halogenation	Y/N	
Chlorine		
Bromine		
Recorder		

WHIRLPOOL SPAS

Halogenation	No.	Location (Deck #)
Chlorine		
Bromine		
Recorder		

SPA/POOL

Halogenation	No.	Location (Deck #)
Chlorine		
Bromine		
Recorder		

Miscellaneous

	Number	Location (Deck #)
Children's Areas		
Activity Center		
Care Center		
Decorative Fountains		
Housekeeping		
Handwash Stations		
Ventilation Units	Y/N	
ACCESSIBLE		

www.ingramcontent.com/pod-product-compliance
Lightning Source LLC
Chambersburg PA
CBHW080302180526
45167CB00006B/2635